H.T. Lutz · H.A. Gharbi

Manual of Diagnostic Ultrasound in Infectious Tropical Diseases

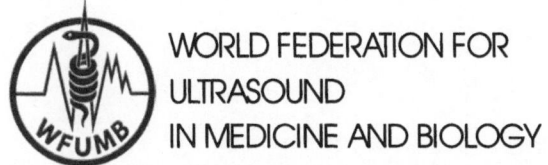

WORLD FEDERATION FOR
ULTRASOUND
IN MEDICINE AND BIOLOGY

Harald T. Lutz
Hassen A. Gharbi
(Editors)

Manual of Diagnostic Ultrasound in Infectious Tropical Diseases

With 176 Figures and 10 Tables

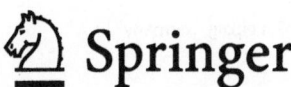 Springer

Prof. Harald T. Lutz
Klinikum Bayreuth
95445 Bayreuth
Germany

Dr. Hassen A. Gharbi
Radiology Department Ibn Zohr
Route X2, Cité El Khadra
Tunis 1003
Tunisia

Library of Congress Control Number: 2005927419

ISBN-10 3-540-24446-8 Springer Berlin Heidelberg New York
ISBN-13 978-3-540-24446-2 Springer Berlin Heidelberg New York

Springer is a part of Springer Science+Business Media
springeronline.com
© Springer-Verlag Berlin Heidelberg 2006

Editor: Dr. Ute Heilmann, Heidelberg
Desk Editor: Wilma McHugh, Heidelberg
Cover design: Frido Steinen-Broo, EStudio Calamar, Spain
Typesetting and production: LE-TeX Jelonek, Schmidt & Vöckler GbR, Leipzig, Germany
Printed on acid-free paper   21/3152/YL – 5 4 3 2 1 0

Foreword

It is with great pleasure and pride that the World Federation for Ultrasound in Medicine and Biology (WFUMB) publishes this "Manual of Diagnostic Ultrasound in Infectious and Tropical Diseases". This is a book that will satisfy a great need that up to now has been unfulfilled. Although there are many books that deal with various aspects of ultrasound, this is the only one that deals specifically with infectious and tropical diseases. It will provide much-needed knowledge and insight in these areas. It will be of especially great value in the teaching of health professionals in those parts of the world where ultrasound is just beginning to be incorporated into patient care.

This book has had the good fortune to be conceived and edited by Drs. Lutz and Gharbi. They are excellent physician practitioners of ultrasound with much experience in teaching in the developing world. They have gathered together an outstanding array of chapter authors to create a most valuable book. All of the authors are to be congratulated on a job well done.

I trust that readers of this book will benefit from the material contained and will be enabled to provide better medical care to their patients. This is certainly a worthy aim, and one that WFUMB is constantly working to achieve.

Marvin C. Ziskin, M.D.
President, WFUMB

Preface

Diagnostic ultrasound is a rapidly developing imaging technology widely used in both industrialized and developing countries, as stated by a WHO Study Group in 1996. Ultrasound is especially suitable for poorer countries even outside the centers of population, since ultrasound does not need a sophisticated infrastructure or expensive installations, but can be used with transportable units even without a direct branch connection. Ultrasound can be used not only as really universal diagnostic method but also as a suitable guide for simple and careful therapeutic interventions, not at least in infectious and parasitic diseases, such as bilharziosis, amebiasis or hydatid disease. The method is safe concerning the bioeffects, but the safety of a diagnostic tool also depends on the accuracy of the results, i.e., on the experience and the skill of the persons using the equipment.

Therefore the World Federation of Ultrasound in Medicine and Biology (WFUMB) is focusing upon (biological) safety and upon education as well, in cooperation with the WHO.

The stimulus to publish this small manual came from an African colleague during an ultrasound course organized by the WFUMB. He said there existed a number of nice and suitable manuals and books about ultrasound in general, but he had not found a small manual dealing with the specific infectious diseases common in subtropical and tropical regions.

Following his proposal, we set out to design a small manual on these topics, not for the big libraries, but for direct use during the examination. It should help our colleagues working in these areas and should encourage them to use ultrasound on a large scale, including interventional ultrasound, for the benefit of their patients.

For us it was really a great experience to find that all our colleagues, individual members of the WFUMB from all parts of the world, agreed without reservation to cooperate in writing this manual. We really do hope that it was possible to distill the long experience of all these colleagues in this small manual. At the same time, we recognize that this was a first attempt. Therefore, we invite all colleagues to help us to eradicate mistakes and further improve the manual in the future.

Harald T. Lutz
Hassen A. Gharbi

Acknowledgements

The editors would like to thank Drs. R. Badea, Cluj-Napoca, Romania, Gertrud Jechart, Augsburg, Germany and Gebhard Mathis, Hohenems, Austria for the courteousness to support us with interesting images.

The editors thank all the colleagues in the board of the WFUMB for encouraging, supporting and advising us, during the preparation of the manual.

The editors express their special appreciation of the valuable and selfless help of Peter N.T. Wells. With his great experience as editor in chief of the official journal UMB of the WFUMB, he checked the manuscripts arriving from the different parts of the world very carefully and gave us many useful and good advice.

Harald T. Lutz
Hassen A. Gharbi

Acknowledgements

Contents

List of Contributors

Fernando Amaral
MEDIAX
Memorial Imagem e Diagnostico
Recife, Brazil

Alfonso Julio G. Barbato
University of Sao Paulo
Sao Paulo, Brazil

Nestor de Barros
School of Medicine
University of Sao Paulo
Sao Paulo, Brazil

Ibtissem Bellagha
Radiology Department
Children's Hospital
Place Bab Sardoun
Tunis Jabbari,
1007 Tunisia

Alessandra Caremani
Department of Infectious Disease
San Donato Hospital
Arezzo, Italy

Marcello Caremani
Department of Infectious Disease
San Donato Hospital
Arezzo, Italy

Giovanni Guido Cerri
School of Medicine
University of Sao Paulo
Sao Paulo, Brazil

Maria Cristina Chammas
School of Medicine
University of Sao Paulo
Sao Paulo, Brazil

Ferid Ben Chehida
Radiology Department Ibn Zohr
Route X2, Cité El Khadra
Tunis 1003, Tunisia

Michel Claudon
Department of Radiology
University of Nancy
France

Josef Deuerling
Klinikum Bayreuth
Bayreuth, Germany

Wiem Douira
Radiology Department
Children's Hospital
Place Bab Sardoun
Tunis Jabbari,
1007 Tunisia

Gerusa Dreyer
Núcleo de Ensino Pesquisa
e Assistencia em Filariose (NEPAF)
Hospital das Clinicas
Av. Prof. Moraes Rego s/n
Cidade Universitária
Recife PE, 50740–900, Brazil

Leandro J. Fernandez
Director, Laboratory
of Advanced Ultrasound
La Floresta Medical Institute
Caracas, Venezuela

Alain Gerard
Department of Tropical Diseases
University of Nancy
France

Hassen A. Gharbi
Radiology Department Ibn Zohr
Route X2, Cité El Khadra
Tunis 1003, Tunisia

Azza Hammou
Centre National
de Radio-protection
Bab Saadoun
Tunis 1007 Jebbari, Tunisia

Joon-Koo Han
Seoul National University
College of Medicine
28 Yongon-Dong, Chongno-Gu
Seoul 110–744, Korea

Nathan Herszkowicz
School of Medicine
University of Sao Paulo
Sao Paulo, Brazil

Mohammed Salah Kechaou
Department of Radiology
Habib Bourguiba Hospital,
Sfax, Tunisia

Harald T. Lutz
Klinikum Bayreuth
Bayreuth, Germany

Alix Martin-Bertaux
Department of Radiology
University of Nancy
France

Sana Mezghani
Department of Radiology
Habib Bourguiba Hospital
Sfax, Tunisia

Jamel Mnif
Department of Radiology
Habib Bourguiba Hospital
Sfax, Tunisia

Zeineb Mnif
Department of Radiology
Habib Bourguiba Hospital
Sfax, Tunisia

Joaquim Noroes
Dept de Parasitologia Pesquisas,
Centro Aggeu
Magalhâes-Fiocruz,
Recife, Brazil

Ilka Regina Souza de Oliveira
School of Medicine
University of Sao Paulo
Sao Paulo, Brazil

Heykel Ben Romdhane
Radiology Department Ibn Zohr
Route X2, Cité El Khadra
Tunis 1003, Tunisia

Waldir Salvi
School of Medicine

University of Sao Paulo
Sao Paulo, Brazil

Danilo Tacconi
Department of Infectious Disease
San Donato Hospital
Arezzo, Italy

CHAPTER 1

Basics of Ultrasound

HARALD T. LUTZ

1.1
Physical and Technical Principals

Ultrasound is the term applied to mechanical pressure waves with frequencies above 20,000 Hz (beyond the audible range).

A medium must be present for ultrasound propagation to occur. In biological tissues, ultrasonic energy is propagated mainly in the form of longitudinal waves, as it is in fluid.

The ultrasound wave can be both emitted and received by a piezoelectric transducer. The piezoelectric transducer is able to change electrical signals into mechanical waves, that is, transmitting ultrasound (= reverse piezoelectric effect), and vice versa to change mechanical pressure (reflected ultrasound waves, "echoes") into electrical signals (= direct piezoelectric effect).

Ultrasound in the MHz range (high-frequency) can be emitted as a directional beam, comparable to a light beam, from transducers of practical size.

Ultrasound waves propagate in biological tissue at an average speed of 1540 meters (m) per second, with the exception of bones, where the waves move at more than 3000 m per second.

Ultrasound waves interact with biological tissue in various ways; they are partially absorbed by the tissue, which means that their energy is converted into heat. This is important for safety reasons (see Sect. 1.5 below). Ultrasound waves can also be reflected (interference > beam diameter) or (back-) scattered on their way through the tissue. Whether reflected or back-scattered, echoes are received by the transducer. These echoes are the source of the diagnostic information.

The echoes are analyzed first with regard to their site of origin (time-distance principle), and secondly with regard to their intensity. This information is used for example to construct an image (two-dimensional

B-scan technique). One of the preconditions is that only a small part of the ultrasound is reflected at each interface, and most of the ultrasound is transmitted to deeper levels. Only bones, gas, and foreign bodies (metallic or nonmetallic) cause a very strong reflection (acoustic shadow); thus no information is obtainable from regions behind such obstacles.

Absorption, reflection, and scattering cause a permanent attenuation of ultrasound energy of approx. 1 decibel per cm of propagation in the tissue traversed per 1 MHz of frequency. The ultrasound attenuation must be corrected by amplifying echoes as a function of distance from the transducer (TGC), in order to get a homogeneous display of the echoes (Fig. 1.1a–d). Nevertheless this attenuation can seriously limit the depth

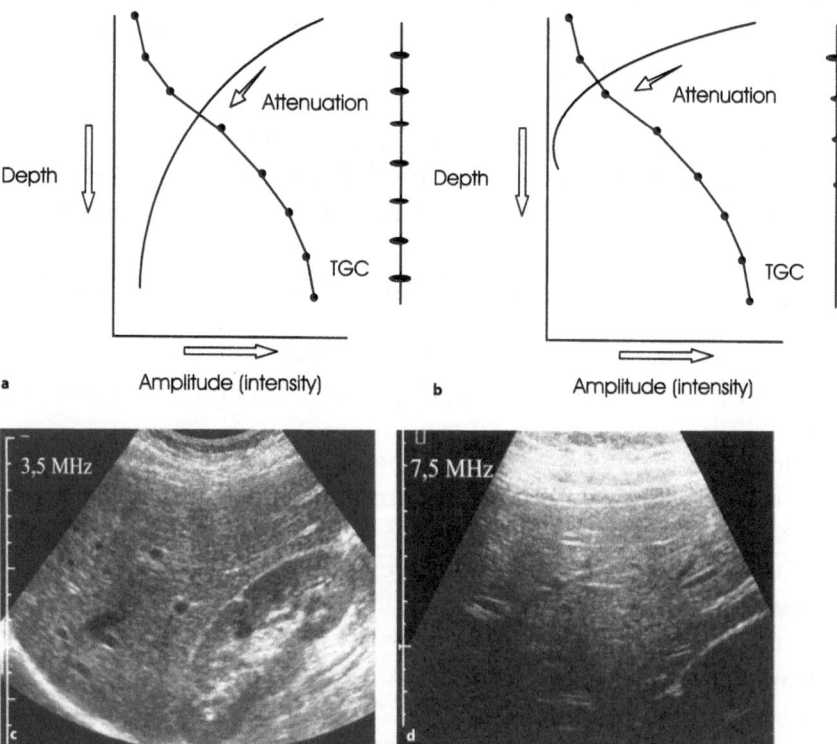

Fig. 1.1a–d. Ultrasound attenuation in the tissue and its correction by the TGC. With 3.5 MHz, a homogeneous image is possible (**a,c**), whereas a frequency of 7.5 MHz (**b,d**) is too high for the examination of the abdomen. On the other side, the resolution close to the 7.5-MHz transducer is better (small-part transducer)

of penetration of higher frequencies (the so-called small part transducers are suitable for small *and superficial* organs only!).

The *ultrasonic field* is a geometric description of the region encompassed by the ultrasound beam. There are two main sectors, the near field (interference field), located between the ultrasound transducer and the (natural) focus, and the far field. The lateral boundary of the ultrasound field is not sharp, because the beam intensity falls off continuously with distance from the center (Fig. 1.2).

The *lateral resolution* depends on the diameter of the ultrasound beam: the smaller the diameter, the better the resolution. The resolution therefore is best in the focal area. The ultrasound beams are focused (mainly electronically by modern techniques), enabling the clinician to always focus on the region of interest (Fig. 1.3).

The *axial resolution* depends on the length of the emitted ultrasound pulses and finally on the wave length, i.e., the frequency.

These basic physical principles are still important in regard to the quality of ultrasound equipment despite the advances in electronic techniques:

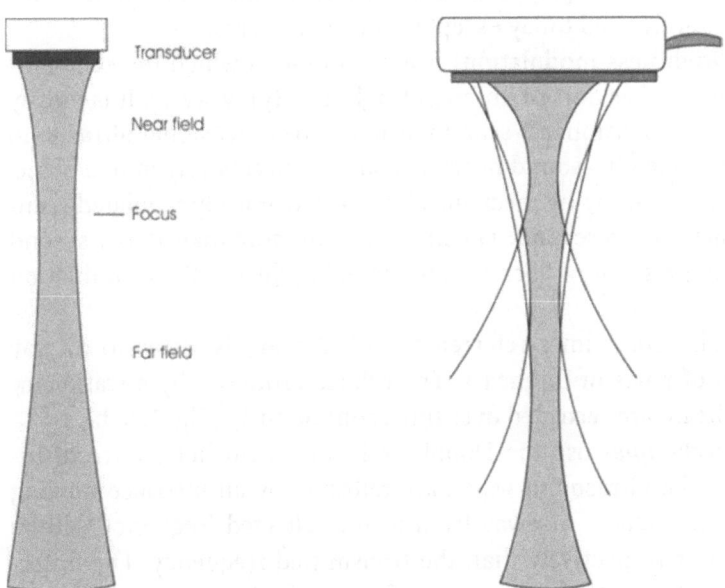

Fig. 1.2. The ultrasonic field of a flat transducer

Fig. 1.3. Schematic representation of electronic focusing of a linear array transducer

the higher the frequency, the better the resolution on the one hand, but the higher the attenuation in the tissue on the other hand, which means a limited penetration depth. For small and superficial parts, therefore, high-frequency transducers (5–10 MHz) should be used, whereas for the abdomen or in late pregnancy, transducers with lower frequencies (2–5 MHz) are necessary.

1.2
Imaging Techniques

The echo principle forms the basis of all of the commonly used diagnostic ultrasound techniques. These are:

A-scan
M-scan
B-scan
Doppler techniques

A-scan (amplitude modulation) is a one-dimensional technique. The echoes received are displayed on a screen as vertical deflections. This technique is rarely used today except for measurements.

B-scan (brightness modulation) is a technique in which the echo amplitude is depicted as dots of different brightness (gray scale). It is mostly used as a two-dimensional B-scan to form a two-dimensional ultrasound image by multiple ultrasound beams, arranged successively in one plane. The images are built up by mechanically or electronically regulated scanning in a fraction of a second. The image rate of more than 15 per second enables an impression of "permanent" imaging during the examination (real time).

M-scan (also sometimes referred to as TM-scan) is a way to display motion, e.g. of parts of the heart. The echoes produced by a stationary ultrasound beam are recorded over time, continuously (Fig. 1.4a,b).

Doppler techniques use the Doppler effect as a further source of information: if the ultrasound waves are reflected by an interface moving towards the transducer or away from it, the reflected frequency will be higher or lower respectively than the transmitted frequency. The difference between the emitted and received frequencies is proportional to the speed of the moving reflector. This phenomenon is called the Doppler effect, and the difference is called the Doppler frequency or Doppler shift.

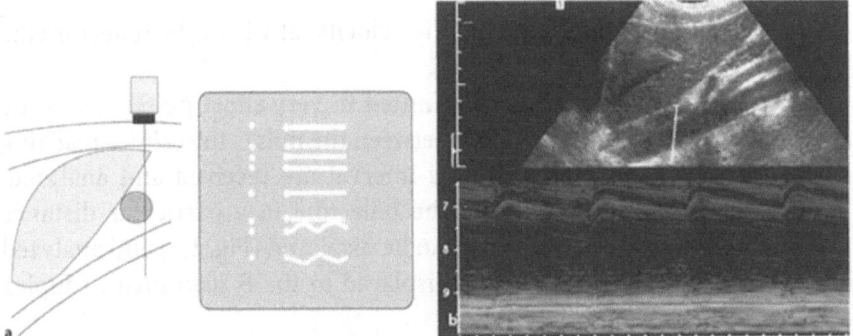

Fig. 1.4. M-scan. Schematic representation (**a**) and original image (**b**). Note the movement of the wall of the aorta. The *line* in the B-scan image marks the area of the M-scan

The Doppler shift depends on the ultrasonic frequency (f), the velocity of the reflector (v), and the angle between the ultrasound beam and the blood stream. Information can only achieved if the angle is less than 60°. An angle of 90° has the cosine $\alpha = 0$, which means no Doppler shift = no signal.

Doppler Formula: $\Delta f = 2f/c \cdot v \cdot \cos\ \alpha$.

There are various Doppler techniques:

- *Continuous wave Doppler* (cw Doppler): the transducer is divided in two parts: one crystal transmits ultrasound permanently, the other crystal receives all the echoes. There is no information about the distance of

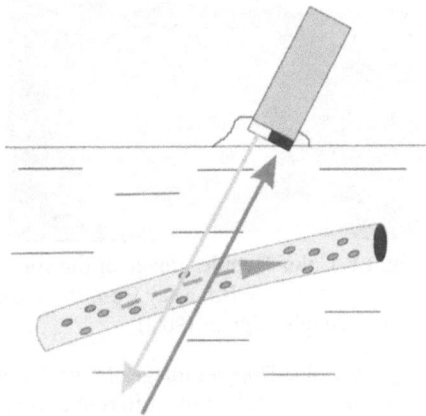

Fig. 1.5. Diagram of the cw Doppler technique. Note the two crystals

the reflector(s), but only about the velocity, at which the reflector (the blood stream) moves (Fig. 1.5).

– *Pulsed Doppler*: Ultrasound is emitted in very short pulses (as in the A-,B-, and M-scan techniques). Between the pulses the echoes reaching the transducer in a certain time interval are received and analyzed. In this way, the movement of the reflectors in a particular distance (gate, selected by the operator) can be displayed (Fig. 1.6) and analyzed (spectral Doppler, Fig. 1.7), or displayed in the B-scan image (duplex techniques, Figs. 1.8–1.10).

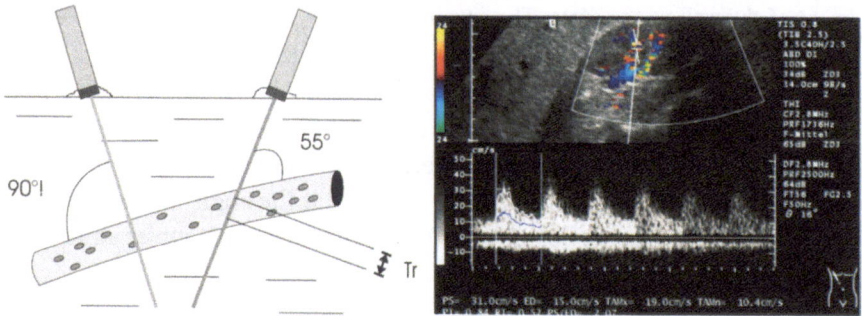

Fig. 1.6. Pulsed Doppler. The echoes, received in a definite time distance (so-called sample volume), are analyzed (in this example marked with "Tr"). The ultrasound beam of the left transducer crosses the vessel at a 90° angle; this means no Doppler signal, as is demonstrated in Fig. 1.8

Fig. 1.7. Spectral Doppler analysis of a segmental artery in the left kidney

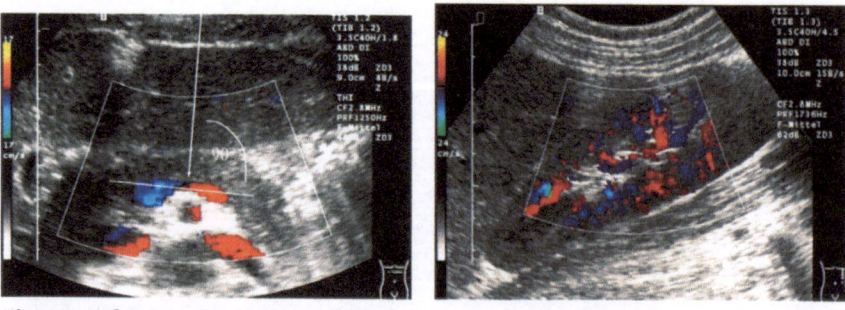

Fig. 1.8. Color-Doppler image of the splenic vein. Flow towards the transducer in the distal part, *red-coded*; away from the transducer in the proximal part, *blue*. Note the gap of Doppler signals (90°!)

Fig. 1.9. Color-Doppler image of the left kidney. The *color-coded* information about the flow direction enables the differentiation between veins and arteries

Fig. 1.10. Power-Doppler image of the right kidney. This technique is more sensitive. In this case it enables the diagnosis of a renal infarction (O)

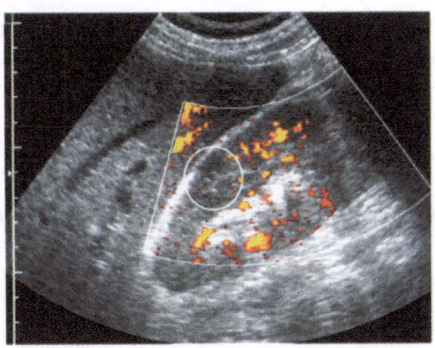

- *Color-Doppler* and *power-Doppler* techniques are used as duplex techniques integrated in the B-scan image. The echoes arising from stationary reflectors (tissue) are displayed as bright spots (gray-scale technique).The echoes from moving reflectors are analyzed by the Doppler technique separately, but displayed in the same image "color-coded". Color-Doppler imaging is based on the mean Doppler frequency shift of the scatterers. The different colors indicate the direction of the blood flow (color-Doppler, CD) (Figs. 1.8, 1.9). Disadvantages of this technique are the angle dependency, especially in the abdomen, and the aliasing artifact.
- The power Doppler technique (synonyms: color Doppler energy or, not as suitable, "ultrasound angiography") is based on the total integrated power of the Doppler signal. This Doppler technique is more sensitive for the detection of small vessels and slow flow and is angle-independent, but does not give information about the direction of the flow (Fig. 1.10).

Contrast agents were originally developed and used to obtain a stronger signal from blood flows. So-called microbubbles, more or less stabilized encapsulated gas bubbles, somewhat smaller than erythrocytes, are used for this purpose. The use of these contrast agents considerably improves the visibility of small vessels with slow flow. However, the real advantage is the possibility to get more detailed information about the static and especially the dynamic vascularity of tissues and tumors. Special software programs and efficient equipment are necessary to use this interesting technique, including, for example, contrast harmonic imaging. With this technique the nonlinear interaction of the microbubbles with ultrasound power is used, to improve the Doppler signals. This new tech-

nique improves the quality of ultrasound in a way similar to that seen
with the tissue harmonic imaging technique used for the B-mode (see
Fig. 2.16).

1.3
General Remarks and Recommendations on Examination Technique

1.3.1
Applications

All body regions which are not situated behind bones or gas-containing
tissues (lung!) are accessible to ultrasonic examination. However, even the
periosteum and the surface of bones can be demonstrated, e.g. to diagnose
fractured ribs or periosteal abscesses and tumors if the integrity of the
bone is compromised.

1.3.2
Preparation

Preparations for ultrasound examinations depend on the organ or the
region to be examined. No special preparation is needed in many situations, an important advantage of ultrasound compared to other imaging
modalities.

Overlying bowel gas may be an obstacle for scanning the abdomen by
causing a total reflection of the ultrasound. Parts of the pancreas and other
dorsally situated structures cannot be visualized, because they are located
in the acoustic shadow of the gas-containing bowel. To avoid this problem
the following preparations and tricks are recommended:

- examining the patient in a fasting state
- imposing dietary restrictions (avoidance of gas-producing foods)
- physical exercise (walking for 30 min before the examination)
- water contrast (fill up the stomach as an acoustic window to the pancreas
  or the urinary bladder for examination of the small pelvis)
- the water contrast method is also very suitable for demonstrating the
  wall of hollow organs such as the bladder, gall bladder, and stomach.
- Special positioning (see below)

Precaution:
When carrying out ultrasound examinations one must pay attention to the possibility of transmitting infectious material with the transducer or the jelly on the instruments from one patient to another. The transducer and other parts having direct contact with the patient must therefore be cleaned after each examination. The minimum requirements are to wipe off the transducer after each examination and to clean it with a suitable disinfectant agent each day and after the examination of an obviously infectious patient.

A suitable method in infectious patients, and especially in patients with open wounds or other skin lesions, is to slip a disposable glove over the transducer with some jelly on the active surface. The same method with a sterile glove is suitable for ultrasonically guided punctures.

1.3.3
Positioning

Usually the examination is carried out with the patient in supine position. Additional scans in the lateral decubitus and prone positions may be necessary and useful in some situations, especially in obese patients or patients with skeletal deformations. The following positions may be helpful for special examinations:

- hyperextension of the neck for scanning the thyroid gland
- upright position for the evaluation of the pancreas
- prone position for the kidneys, especially the left one
- turning 45° to the left to evaluate the hilus of the liver, the common bile duct, and the head of the pancreas
- pelvic elevation to scan the small pelvis.

1.3.4
Coupling Agents

A coupling agent is necessary to ensure good acoustic contact between the transducer and the skin. Water is not ideal and is useful only for very short examinations. Disinfectant fluids can be used for short contact with the transducer, especially for guided punctures. Oil has the disadvantage of dissolving rubber or plastic parts of the transducer.

Table 1.1. A commonly used formula for a coupling agent for ultrasound

---

Carbomer 10.0 g
EDTA 0.25 g
Propylene glycol 75.0 g
Trolamine 12.5 g
Demineralized water up to 500 ml

Preparation: first combine the EDTA with 400 ml of water. When the EDTA has dissolved, add the propylene glycol. Then add the carbomer to the solution and stir, if possible with a high-speed stirrer, until the mixture forms a gel without bubbles. Add water up to 500 g of gel. Stir carefully to avoid air bubbles.

The best coupling agent is a water-soluble gel, available commercially or homemade (Table 1.1).

1.3.5
General Recommendations and Guidelines for Ultrasound Examinations (Twelve Golden Rules)

Ultrasound examinations must be done by trained people! In addition, the following 12 'Golden Rules' should be respected:

- know the history and the problems of the patient
- make sure that the settings of the equipment are correct
- conduct a systematic examination of the body region of interest, even with obvious palpable mass or circumscribed pain
- always proceed from the known to the unknown, e.g. from the anatomically constant area to a more variable area (e.g. abdomen: start with the liver and proceed to the region of the pancreas or the intestine)
- move the transducer in a slow constant pattern while maintaining the defined scanning plane, and hold the transducer motionless during movements of the patient (respiration)
- use anatomically constant and easily visualized structures for orientation (e.g. liver, aorta, fluid-filled bladder) and use normal structures for comparison (right and left kidney, liver parenchyma and kidney)
- demonstrate each organ or mass in at least two planes
- never overlook the possibility of false positive or negative results due to artifacts
- utilize palpation to displace fluid- or gas filled-bowel, to test the consistency of tumors and organs, and to localize points of pain

- continue the entire examination even if pathologies are found early in the exam
- check equipment settings again if findings are questionable
- repeat the examination within a short time in clinically difficult situations

1.4
Interventional Ultrasound

In principle, all percutaneous punctures in body regions accessible to ultrasound examination can be performed using ultrasound guidance. This method is used for the safe puncture of fluid in the various cavities, as for pleural or pericardial effusion or ascites as well as for biopsy of organs such as the liver or kidney or for amniocentesis.

The fine-needle aspiration biopsy in the strict sense was developed for the puncture of suspected tumors in parenchymatous organs and other suspicious masses. The same technique is suitable for the diagnostic puncture of fluid collections in organs or body cavities. These techniques were developed for the treatment of those lesions as well: emptying fluid collections, especially abscesses (if necessary repeatedly), insertion of drains, and application of drugs into parasitic cysts (PAIR) or tumors. Ultrasound has proven to be a nearly ideal puncture guide that has made "classic" percutaneous puncture procedures safer and enabled the development of new diagnostic and therapeutic puncture procedures.

> **Precautions:**
> Interventional procedures should be carried out only by well trained and experienced doctors!
> The ultrasonic-guided punctures are invasive techniques. The puncture must therefore be carried out only if it is clearly indicated. The patient must be informed about this intervention. The puncture must be performed carefully and under strictly sterile conditions.

Coagulation parameters should be checked, at least if any suspicion of hypocoagulability is apparent from the case history.

Fine needles with a diameters less than 1 mm should be used for the diagnostic puncture of (suspected) tumors. It must be remembered that cutting needles are more traumatic than the needles with the same diameter used for aspiration cytology.

The puncture of pheochromocytomas and aneurysms must be avoided.

The puncture of hydatid cysts requires a special technique that must be taken into consideration whenever a cystic lesion should be punctured (see Chap. 3, Sect. 3.3.7.1).

The best needle route is selected by ultrasound, and the puncture tract should be free of large vessels and other problematic structures. However, it is not a problem to puncture through the gastrointestinal tract or the bladder with thin needles, since the walls of these organs contain muscular fibers.

The transpulmonary route should be avoided when puncturing the abdomen.

When puncturing superficial lymph nodes, and especially if tuberculosis is suspected, it is useful to shift the skin over the lymph node, to avoid the development of fistulas.

1.4.1
Technique

The technique described here pertains to fine-needle aspiration but is conceptually valid for other types of percutaneous puncture as well.

The skin is cleaned carefully with a disinfecting solution and infiltrated with a local anesthetic.

The exact procedure depends on the type of ultrasound system used, especially whether or not special biopsy transducers are used.

Special biopsy transducers combined with a suitable software program make the puncture easier. They are necessary if small and distant targets should be punctured. The disadvantages of these convenient techniques are the higher expenses. Not only is a special transducer needed in the beginning, but also more expensive special (disposable) needles must be used. Furthermore, the biopsy transducer must be sterilized or enveloped in a sterile cover.

The so-called free-hand puncture is a more primitive method, but needs less "infrastructure". No special needles are necessary, and the normal transducer used need not be sterilized.

In this technique, the most favorable puncture site is first marked on the skin in two planes during the ultrasound examination. The distance between the surface of the skin and the target can be measured on the screen and marked on the needle, if necessary. The direction of the needle insertion corresponds to the direction of the scan. The transducer will

Fig. 1.11. Free-hand puncture of ascites. The position of the needle is demonstrated by the transducer placed at the side

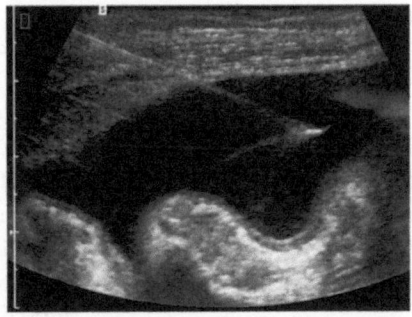

be removed and the puncture will be carried out after having the skin disinfected. The correct position of the needle tip in the target can be controlled with the transducer from the side (Fig. 1.11).

For the diagnostic puncture of fluid collections and for the fine-needle aspiration cytology of suspected tumors, no special needles are necessary. Only if the puncture of a suspected tumor is being performed to get histological samples are special (and much more expensive) needle systems required.

1.4.2
Evaluation of the Aspirated Material

1.4.2.1
Fluid (Cystic Lesions)

The evaluation of the aspirated fluid is based on its appearance, some simple laboratory tests, and on bacteriological examinations if an infectious disease is suspected (Tables 1.2, 1.3). In this case, aerobic and anaerobic cultures are ideal, but for a first orientation, staining methods are suitable (e.g. methylene blue or Gram's staining method).

If a microscopic examination of cells in the aspirated fluid is necessary, the material should be centrifuged and prepared immediately to avoid destruction of the cells.

1.4.2.2
Solid Lesion

For cytological examination, the lesion should be punctured in a fan-like pattern in order to obtain representative material. Drops of the aspirated

Table 1.2. Appearance of fluid

Clear, transparent, light-yellow	Serous exudate
Clear like water	Hydatid cyst
Opaque, fine clots	Fibrinous exudate
cloudy-purulent (smell)	Exudate with leukocytes, empyema, abscess
Milky	Chylous fluid
Homogeneous bright–dark red	Sanguinolent, fresh – old blood
Bright red veils	Fresh blood admixture caused by the puncture procedure
Dark green–brown	Amoebic (liver) abscess

Table 1.3. Simple laboratory tests for the differentiation of aspirated fluid

Specific gravity > 1015	Exudate
Protein elevated	Exudate
Moritz-Rivalta-probe (acetic acid) positive	Exudate
Creatine elevated	Urine
Amylase	Pancreatic ascites or pseudocyst
Bilirubin	Biloma
Cholesterol elevated (> 50 mg/dl)	Malignant

material in the syringe are brought on microscopic slides and spread in a thin film with a second glass placed over the first slide or with the needle itself. The specimens are air-dried or wet-fixed or a spray fixative is used, following the recommendations of the person who will analyze the material. To obtain histological specimens, special fine "cutting" needles are used.

The puncture should not be aimed at the center of (larger) lesions, in order to avoid the biopsy of necrotic material.

1.4.2.3
Therapeutic Puncture of Fluid Collections

If with a diagnostic puncture purulent fluid is aspirated – which means that the diagnosis of an abscess or an empyema, respectively, is established – the procedure can be expanded as an appropriate treatment. In a first step, the abscess is emptied as far as possible. Sometimes a thicker needle (1.2 mm) is needed. Irrigation with saline is helpful for this purpose.

The success of the treatment is controlled with ultrasound over the next few days. Often a single puncture with emptying of at least 80% of the abscess is sufficient, and the abscess heals under continued antibiotic therapy. In other cases, the procedure must be repeated after 2–3 days. Alternatively, a catheter of suitable caliber (depending on the viscosity of the pus) is introduced under ultrasonic guidance, using, for example, the Seldinger technique. The correct position of the catheter is normally controlled by ultrasound. The catheter is irrigated each day and can also be used for the local instillation of antibiotics until the abscess disappears and the cavity has collapsed.

1.4.3
Hazards

Percutaneous punctures are contraindicated by coagulation disorders. If the coagulation is normal, the fine-needle puncture of tumors has a very low risk of serious hemorrhage. The risk becomes much higher if thicker needles are used (Fig. 1.12.).

The danger of introducing tumor cells into the needle track has been studied by many authors. Single cases of inoculation metastases have been described. However, based on extensive experience and many studies, this risk seems to be so small that generally it does not represent a contraindication. Much more so, this technique seems to be the less risky method to establish a final diagnosis in many cases.

The risk of spreading infectious material has also been extensively discussed and studied. The method has proven to be very useful for the treatment of abscesses and other pyogenic lesions. Nevertheless, in some special parasitic diseases, the risk of spreading a living organism must be

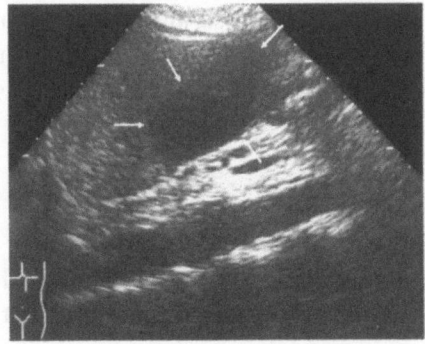

Fig. 1.12. Hemorrhage after fine-needle puncture of the liver. The hemorrhage of around 70 ml (measured with ultrasound) in this case was unusual, but did not need any treatment

considered carefully. A typical example of this problem is echinococcosis (see Chap. 3, Sect. 3.3.7.1).

1.5
Safety
(by Hassen A. Gharbi, Heykel Ben Romdhane, Azza Hammou, Férid Ben Chehida, Ibtissem Bellagha)

Physicians have used ultrasound to make images of the inside of the human body for nearly half a century. Around the world, with the exception of some areas affected by poverty, most of the infants born within recent times were exposed to ultrasound before birth. In some countries, all pregnant women are screened with ultrasound. To date, researchers around the world have not identified any adverse biological effects clearly caused by ultrasound used in medical fields. This is an enviable safety record.

However, all of the experts around the world advocate continued study of ultrasound safety, improvements in the safety features of ultrasound, and more safety education for ultrasound system operators. In light of the sheer numbers of people exposed to ultrasound, any possibility of a harmful effect must be investigated thoroughly.

1.5.1
Ultrasound Effects

While it remains unclear whether there are any long-term effects of the diagnostic ultrasound in use today, scientists do know from laboratory studies and from industrial use of ultrasound that ultrasound at high intensities does create immediate effects at the time of exposure. From studies in test tubes, animals, and human beings, we know that ultrasound causes heating, referred to as ultrasound's thermal effect. Ultrasound also creates nonthermal effects, also known as mechanical effects.

1.5.1.1
Thermal Effects

As ultrasound waves pass through the body, their energy is partially absorbed and converted into heat, heat absorbed by the tissues of the body.

In general, the more dense the tissue, the more heat is absorbed, as the ultrasound waves cannot pass through dense tissue as easily. Thus fluid does not heat up very much, soft tissues heat up somewhat more, and bone heats up the most.

This thermal effect is used in industries and in laboratories but must be avoided in medical use.

1.5.1.2
Nonthermal Effects

Ultrasound's nonthermal effects include audible sounds, the movement of cells in liquid, electrical changes in cell membranes, shrinking and expansion of bubbles in liquid, and pressure changes. Researching these thermal and nonthermal effects in the laboratory should help scientists to determine which long-term effects to check for in the human population.

In addition to heat, scientists have begun to learn more about the various types of mechanical effects that ultrasound can have on the body. They divide these effects into two categories.

The first category is called acoustic cavitation. Cavitation can occur when sound passes through an area that contains a cavity, such as a gas bubble or other air pocket. Some tissues, most notably adult lung and intestine, do contain air bubbles, and are therefore more vulnerable to these cavitation effects. The fetal lung and intestine do not contain obvious air bubbles, because the fetus does not breath air yet, getting oxygen from the mother's blood stream. However, researchers believe that tiny bubbles could potentially form in parts of the body other than the lung and intestine. More research is needed in this area.

In cavitation, the sound waves can cause the bubbles or air pockets to expand and contract rhythmically; in other words, to pulsate, or resonate. When they pulsate, the bubbles send secondary sound waves off in all directions. These secondary sound waves can actually improve ultrasound images because the secondary waves also reflect back to the transducer, and provide more information. Thus, doctors now sometimes inject artificial bubbles known as ultrasound contrast agents into the body before taking ultrasound images, for instance, for the circulatory system. However, these contrast agents are not used to image the fetus.

Other effects: If the bubbles contract towards the point of collapsing, they can build up very high temperatures and pressures for a few tens of nanoseconds. These high temperatures and high pressures can produce highly reactive chemicals called free radicals and other potentially toxic compounds that, although considered unlikely, could theoretically cause genetic damage. The rapid contraction of bubbles in cavitation can also cause microjets of liquid that can damage cells. When diagnostic ultrasound is focused on the lung or intestine of laboratory animals, which contain gas bubbles, these cavitation effects can cause ruptures in very small blood vessels.

When ultrasound passes through liquid, it causes a type of stirring action called acoustic streaming. As the acoustic pressure of the ultrasound increases, the flow of liquid speeds up. This stirring action, in theory, could occur in fluid-filled parts of a patient's body, such as blood vessels, the bladder, or amniotic sac. In experiments with animals, when streaming of the liquid comes near a solid object, shearing can occur, and this can damage platelets and lead to abnormal blood clotting (thrombosis). It is not clear to what extent this effect occurs in humans exposed to diagnostic ultrasound.

1.5.1.3
Healing with Ultrasound

It should be noted that even before ultrasound became a widespread diagnostic tool, doctors were using it as a therapeutic tool. The fact that ultrasound does have biological effects on the body is clear from its use to promote healing and even to operate on human beings. Ultrasound speeds the healing of bone, although it is not clear why this occurs. Surgeons are also using highly focused ultrasound beams to operate in delicate areas such as the eyes. The focused beam heats up and selectively destroys a minute portion of the tissue. Studying the therapeutic effects of ultrasound could also yield clues to any possible harmful effects of diagnostic ultrasound.

In conclusion, according to researchers, the relevant literature, and the safety committee conclusions of the World Federation of Ultrasound in Medicine and Biology, the use of ultrasound for medical diagnosis does not produce any adverse biological effects. Ultrasound examination is safe and accurate.

However the doctor or technician must respect the following golden rules:

1. Ultrasound examinations must be done only by well-trained clinicians
2. Ultrasound examinations must respect the maximum of energy allowed
3. An ultrasound examinations must be done only when the patient's situation indicates its need. All-over use of ultrasound must be avoided.

CHAPTER 2

Typical Sonographic Findings in Inflammatory Diseases

HARALD T. LUTZ · HASSEN A. GHARBI

In this chapter, the general ultrasonic findings in inflammatory diseases will be discussed, based on the pathologic alterations. The reaction of the body to different pathologic organisms (and other injuries) is rather uniform. Many sonographic findings seen in inflammatory and infectious diseases are rather nonspecific for a certain organism or a certain disease.

These sonographic symptoms are based on the general reactions of living tissue attacked by organisms. Only the clinical background, the localization, or the duration as well as typical complications may enable a more specific diagnosis with ultrasound in some situations.

2.1
Pathology of Inflammation, Common Findings

Injuries of living tissue by organisms (viruses, bacteria, fungi, or parasites) generally cause:

- dilatation of small vessels and increased blood flow (= redness, heat)
- increased permeability, leading to accumulation of interstitial fluid, solute, and protein (= edema, swelling, exudation)
  The type of exudate depends on factors related to the agent and the anatomical location as well:
  - serous exudate (low protein), typical of surfaces outlined with mesothelium
  - fibrinous exudate (high protein), typical of serous-lined cavities
  - purulent exudate, caused by pyogenic agents (empyema in preformed cavities)
  - hemorrhagic exudate, caused by damage of small vessels.

Edemas and exudates may cause complications by loss of functional tissue (e.g., lung tissue) or obstruction.

– emigration of leukocytes, neutrophils, or monocytes (= cellular infiltration)

Abscesses are caused by pyogenic bacteria or parasites in soft tissue and parenchymatous organs. Typical is a liquefied center of necrosis, surrounded by a layer of fibrin and leukocytes, and limited by a wall of fibroblasts, small new vessels, and young collagen fibers (barrier and repair process).

Gangrene: necrotic tissue destroyed by putrefactive microorganisms. Gas gangrene is caused by clostridia producing CO_2, especially in anaerobic conditions.

Lesions caused by parasites may have different features depending on the parasite itself and the tissue affected. In general the lesion is characterized by the appearance of the parasite(s) and the reaction of the host, e.g., granulomas or encapsulation.

In the stage of healing, there may be a complete return to functional and structural normality (resolution), or there may be a replacement of destroyed tissue by scar tissue (repair).

A typical problem in this situation is the organization of (fibrinous) exudate, causing adhesions (e.g., in the abdomen) or obliteration of cavities (pleura).

In other situations, with persistence of the infection or inadequate response of the host, the inflammation may become chronic.

A special type of chronic inflammation is granulomatous inflammation, caused by various organisms, e.g., *Mycobacteria*, *Toxoplasma*, or *Leishmania*. This type is characterized by granulomas consisting of a large number of macrophages, e.g., in the lung or the liver.

2.2
Ultrasonic Findings

Dilatation of the small vessels and hyperemia cannot be demonstrated with Ultrasound B-scan directly, but only by using Doppler techniques. With color Doppler or power Doppler, the hyperemia (e.g., in lymph nodes or in an organ) will be demonstrated more qualitatively (Fig. 2.1). By using the spectral Doppler technique, the increased flow in the feeding artery of an organ can be measured quantitatively.

Edema of soft tissue or organs causes swelling or enlargement, which can be demonstrated and measured in the ultrasonic picture (B-scan) directly.

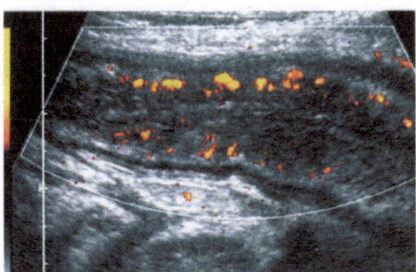 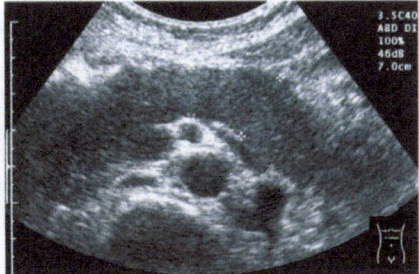

Fig. 2.1. Acute colitis. Segment of the descending colon. Power Doppler shows multiple color pixels in the wall, indicating (inflammatory) hyperemia

Fig. 2.2. Edematous pancreatitis. Note the echo-poor pattern, caused by the inflammatory edema (compare with Fig. 3.13)

The augmented fluid also causes a more echo-poor pattern of the tissue involved. An improved sound transmission may be seen (Fig. 2.2, 2.28, 2.49).

Serous exudates can be seen easily as echo-free areas in the typical cavities involved, as pericardial (Fig. 2.3) or pleural effusion (see Fig. 2.23) as well as ascites (Fig. 2.4). The high protein content of fibrinous exudates may cause a few weak echoes arranged like threads within the fluid. Additionally a fine net of echoes will be seen if the fibrinogen is converted to fibrin (Fig. 2.5). The same finding can be demonstrated in hemorrhagic or purulent fluids, which are rich in protein as well. Furthermore an increasing number of weak echoes can be seen, sometimes a little sedimented (Fig. 2.6). But it must be considered that, for the demonstration of these weak echoes, a sensitive ultrasound equipment is necessary as well as a correct adjustment of the instrument.

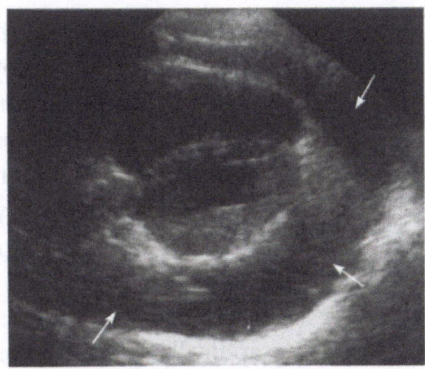

Fig. 2.3. Pericardial effusion (*arrows*)

Fig. 2.4. Serous ascites. The ascites is echo-free. The floating small bowel loops are typical of benign ascites

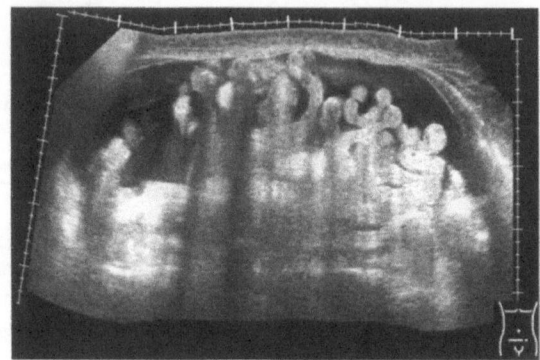

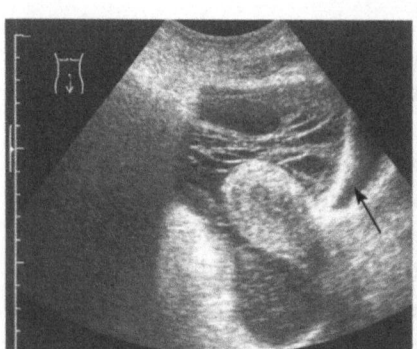

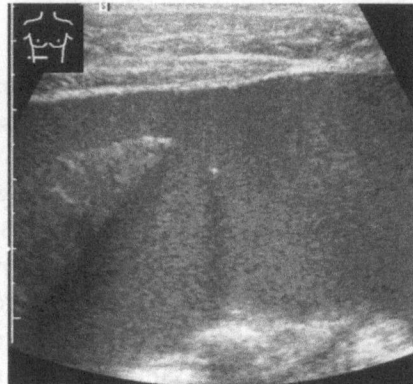

Fig. 2.5. Hemorrhagic ascites. The fibrin in the fluid forms a net of echoes. (Scan through the lower part of the abdomen with the fluid around the uterus. The nearly empty bladder on the right side is marked by an *arrow*)

Fig. 2.6. Purulent ascites. The bright echo with the acoustic shadow close to the edge of the right hepatic lobe is caused by the tip of the (puncture) needle

   The same problems exist, sometimes, for the demonstration of empyemas: empyemas of the pleura cannot always be distinguished from simple pleural effusions by demonstrating echoes within the fluid in general (Fig. 2.7). In the same way, an empyema of the gall bladder does not show inner echoes regularly, whereas, conversely, echoes within the gall bladder may be caused by very small crystals as so-called sludge, indicating a fasting period but not a disorder of the gallbladder (see Figs. 2.42 and 2.43b).
   Abscesses in the soft tissue and in parenchymatous organs are demonstrated sonographically as focal lesions. Three types can be distinguished:

Fig. 2.7. Pleural empyema. Unusual marked finding, with strong echoes indicating gas or air

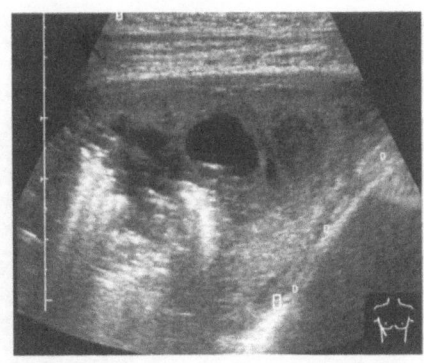

the first type is a nearly echo-free focal lesion, like a cyst (Fig. 2.8, 2.35). Only a more irregular shape and especially the blurred outline may help to distinguish this type from true cysts. The second type is the "tumor-like" type. It shows the character of a solid focal lesion (Figs. 2.9, 2.36). This type cannot be differentiated from a tumor on grounds of the ultrasonic finding alone, but only on the clinical background. The third type shows an irregular and complex pattern, sometimes with some strong echoes indicating gas bubbles. Despite the sometimes confusing picture in the first moment, this type is characteristic of abscesses and does not cause differential diagnostic problems (Fig. 2.10, 2.37).

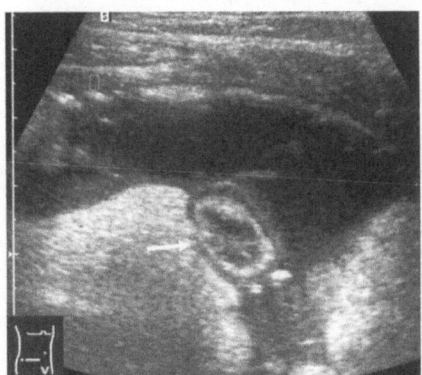
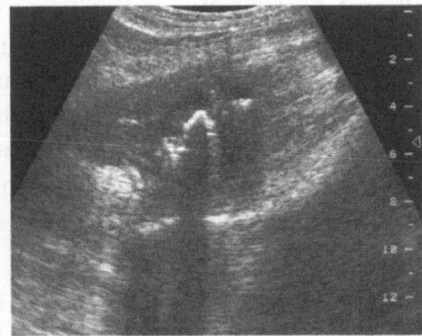

Fig. 2.8. Abscess in the right abdomen, echo-free = type 1. The abscess surrounding the colon (*arrow*) was caused by a perforation of an inborn diverticulum

Fig. 2.9. Psoas abscess, echo-poor = type 2. The strong echo in the center is caused by a foreign body

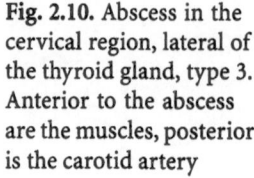

Fig. 2.10. Abscess in the cervical region, lateral of the thyroid gland, type 3. Anterior to the abscess are the muscles, posterior is the carotid artery

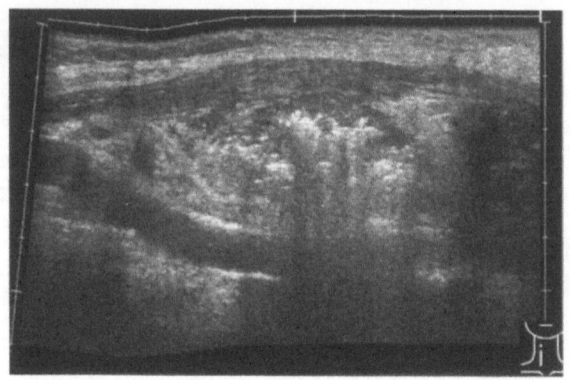

Necrotic tissue and gangrene may show a very variable sonographic pattern, too, depending on the grade of liquefaction and on the presence of gas.

Despite the fact that fluid can easily be demonstrated by ultrasound, the nature of the fluid, serous or purulent, cyst or abscess, cannot be clarified by ultrasound in some situations. For the final diagnosis, a needle puncture is the best way (see Chap. 1, Sect. 1.4). Much more, this method may be not only useful to establish the final diagnosis, but also to treat the infection by emptying the pus or by inserting a drain in the same way. The special problem of parasites, especially hydatid cysts, must be taken into consideration in this connection, in order to avoid complications (see Chap. 3, Sect. 3.3.7).

One of the major advantages of ultrasound is the ability to repeat examinations as often as useful without any harm for the patient. Thus the method is very suitable to monitor the course of alterations demonstrated by ultrasound in the beginning, that is, the course of the infection. The regression of the sonographic findings can be demonstrated, indicating the healing as well as the occurrence of complications, such as malfunctions.

Malfunctions may be caused by organization of persisting exudates (see Fig. 2.27). In the pleural cavity, the pleural obstruction can be detected. In the beginning, the scar may be rather echo-poor like fluid, but without movement if the position of the patient is changed. In the abdomen, adhesions can be diagnosed based on the lack of movement of the bowel against the wall (normally 3–5 cm during breathing).

Generally, the development of a chronic inflammation cannot be diagnosed. In the beginning, the alterations of an organ due to the chronicity

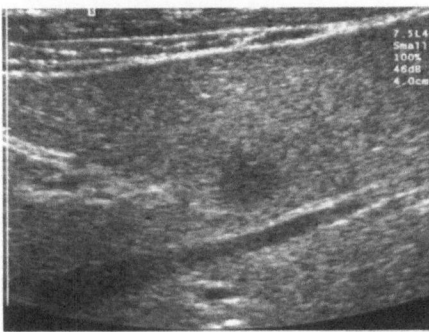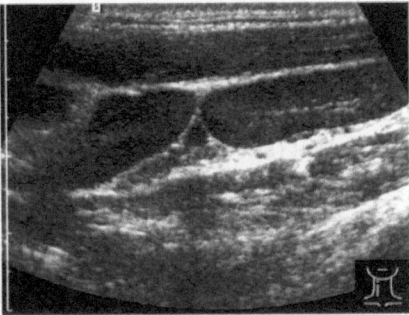

Fig. 2.11. Hepatic granuloma. The relatively large focal lesion with blunt outline is situated in front of the right hepatic vein

Fig. 2.12. Enlarged cervical lymph nodes behind the muscles (M. sternocleidomastoideus) (EBV infection). Note the oval shape and the hilus sign (bright echoes in the center), which indicate a benign disease

of the infection may be very discreet. As a typical example, the development of chronic hepatitis due to viral infection can be seen (see Chap. 3, Sect. 3.2.2, Fig. 3.22). There are no typical sonographic symptoms in the earlier stage of this disease.

The typical granulomas characterizing the granulomatous chronic diseases are, in general, too small to be demonstrated with ultrasound (Figs. 2.11, 2.13). Only the nonspecific enlargement of, e.g., the liver can be seen in such a disease. In some parasitic infections, such as schistosomiasis, they can be demonstrated as hyperechogenic spots in the spleen (see Fig. 3.63).

2.3
Organ-related Ultrasonic Findings

2.3.1
Lymph Nodes

2.3.1.1
Examination Technique

Depending on the location, vessels can be suitable guides to find the lymph nodes. The ultrasound frequency used should be as high as possible.

2.3.1.2
Normal Findings

The size of normal lymph nodes varies from 2 to 15 mm. The shape appears more oval (short axis to long axis ratio, $S:L < 0.5$).

The echo pattern is echo-poor in the periphery, with a more echo-rich pattern in the hilus caused by fatty tissue ("hilus sign"; Fig. 2.12).

With the high-level Doppler technique, the fine-vessel architecture can be demonstrated: signals are seen in the hilus. Vessels are branching out from the hilus ("hilar vascularity"; Fig. 2.14).

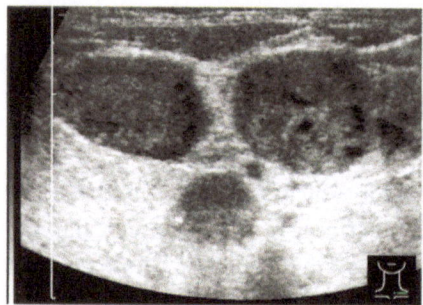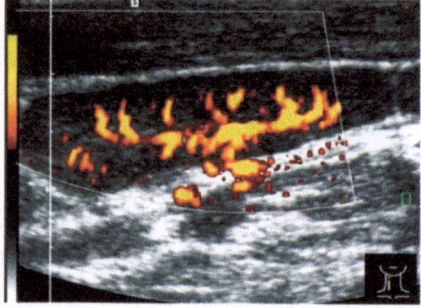

Fig. 2.13. Enlarged cervical lymph nodes (sarcoidosis). Striking are the round shape and the inhomogeneous pattern, caused by small granulomas

Fig. 2.14. Enlarged cervical lymph node (EBV – infection). Power Doppler shows a regular vessel architecture

2.3.1.3
Indications

- palpable (superficial) nodes
- in the neighborhood (lymph drainage) of inflamed tissue and organs
- Toxoplasma
- Tuberculosis
- HIV-related lymphadenopathy

2.3.1.4
Pathologic Findings

Lymph nodes are nearly always involved in inflammatory diseases, either directly by the infectious organism or by draining a local inflammatory region. Typical diseases of the lymph nodes are acute lymphadenitis by pyogenic bacteria, ileocecal yersinial lymphadenitis (Fig. 2.17), infectious mononucleosis, toxoplasmal lymphadenitis, HIV-related lymphadenopathy, and tuberculosis (Table 2.1).

Table 2.1. Typical microorganisms affecting the lymph nodes

Epstein-Barr virus (mononucleosis)

HIV (HIV-related lymphadenopathy)

Pyogenic bacteria, e.g., staphylococci, streptococci (skin, neck)

Yersinia enterocolica, Y. pseudotuberculosis (mesenteric lymphadenitis),

Bartonella henselae (cat-scratch disease)

Mycobacteria (tuberculosis)

Trypanosoma brucei rhodesiense, T. b. gambiense, T. cruzi (trypanomasiasis, Chagas disease)

Toxoplasma gondii (toxoplasmal lymphadenitis)

Wucheria bancroftii (filariasis)

These disorders stimulate different cell populations but do not destroy the architecture of the lymph node at all.

Ultrasonic findings are rather uniform therefore: the lymph nodes involved are enlarged up to 2 cm. Their shape becomes more round and the echo pattern is rather echo-poor. The so-called hilus sign (more echo-rich pattern in the center) still can be demonstrated in most cases (Fig. 2.12). Granulomas (Fig. 2.13) or even caseous degenerations are sometimes too small to be detected by ultrasound, directly. Only tuberculous lymph nodes may show nearly echo-free areas (see Figs. 3.4, 3.5). Abscess formation may be detected if the process penetrates into the surrounding tissue.

The vessel architecture looks quite normal ("hilar vascularity"; Fig. 2.14). But the hyperemia may be conspicuous. Peripheral vascularity, typical of malignant diseases, is described only in tuberculous lymph nodes as well as displacements of vessels.

The resistance index (RI) in inflammatory nodes is generally less than 0.65. Again, in tuberculous nodes, the RI may be higher, up to 0.72.

2.3.1.5
Differential Diagnostic Aspects

The ultrasonic finding of enlarged lymph nodes is not pathognomonic for the type of the disease.

Much more, the differentiation between inflammatory lymph nodes and malignant lymph nodes may be difficult or sometimes even impossible: the malignant lymph nodes are enlarged, but do not always exceed 2 cm. The shape is more round, with a ratio S:L > 0.5, but this is seen in inflammatory nodes as well. The echo pattern is echo-poor, in lymphomas sometimes nearly echo-free. The lack of the hilus sign and an uneven cortex are suspicious for malignant disease as well (Figs. 2.15–2.17).

With color Doppler, a peripheral vascularization (vascular signals on the periphery with branches penetrating into the node) can be demonstrated in metastases, but not always in malignant lymphomas (Fig. 2.16).

The RI is generally higher in malignant diseases, especially metastases (> 0.8).

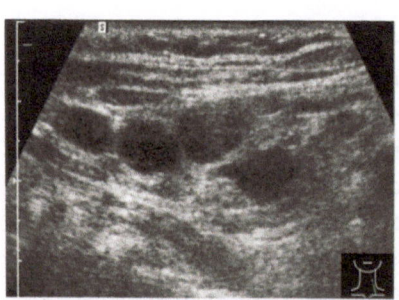 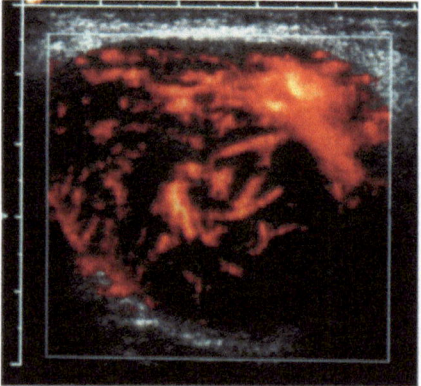

Fig. 2.15. Enlarged cervical lymph nodes. Note the round shape and the lack of the hilus sign: malignant lymphoma (compare with Fig. 2.13)

Fig. 2.16. Enlarged cervical lymph node. Power Doppler shows an irregular vascular architecture: Hodgkin's disease

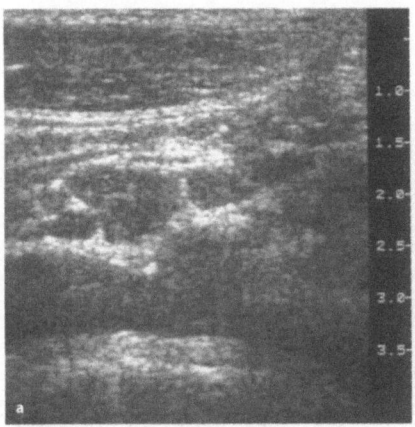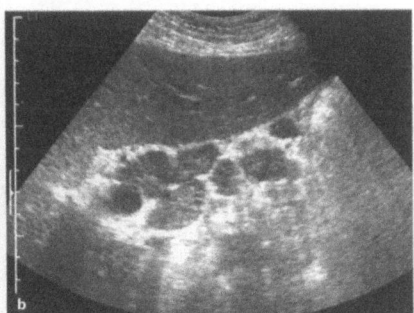

Fig. 2.17. a *Yersinia* lymphadenitis. Enlarged lymph nodes in the ileocecal region, in front of the iliac artery. **b** Malignant lymphoma. Enlarged lymph nodes in the mesentery

Toxoplasma lymphadenitis:
Toxoplasmosis is a worldwide infectious disease caused by the protozoan *Toxoplasma gondii*. Latent symptomless infections are common. This is an important opportunistic infection that may also afflict immunodeficient persons (e.g., those with AIDS, or undergoing chemotherapy).

There are two routes of infection, intrauterine and extrauterine. The congenital toxoplasmosis is mainly a disease of the central nervous system. The latter acquired infection commonly remains latent. Especially in immunodeficient patients, rapid multiorgan involvement may occur.

Lymphadenitis and, more rarely, ophthalmitis are typical manifestations.

The lymph nodes are painless and enlarged due to follicular hyperplasia and small epithelial granulomas.

Ultrasound is able to demonstrate the enlarged lymph nodes, but there is no specific echo-pattern. The spleen may also be enlarged with a homogeneous echo pattern, since the inflammatory foci and granulomas are too small to be seen.

2.3.2
Spleen

2.3.2.1
Examination Technique

- Preparation not required
- Supine or right lateral decubitus
- Longitudinal scans using the lateral approach in different respiratory phases
- Additionally oblique intercostal and subcostal scans
- Measurement: greatest diameter between the diaphragm and the lower "pole"
- Examination should include the demonstration of the splenic artery and vein.

2.3.2.2
Normal Findings

- Maximum dimension 11 × 4 (thickness) cm.
- Echo pattern homogeneous, slightly more echo-dense than the liver. Intrasplenic vessels with B-scan recognizable only close to the hilus (Fig. 2.18).
- Diameter of the splenic vein < 10 mm. Splenic artery: diameter 4–8 mm, mean flow velocity about 30 cm/s with a wide variety, RI < 0.6.
- Typical variation: small accessory spleens, situated mostly close to the hilus (Fig. 2.19).

2.3.2.3
Indications

- systemic inflammatory diseases
- acute and chronic inflammatory diseases affecting organs in the abdomen
- Protozoan infections such as malaria or leishmaniasis
- Chronic liver disease
- Suspicion on portal hypertension

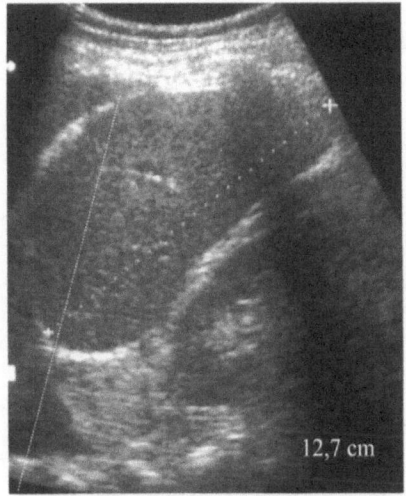 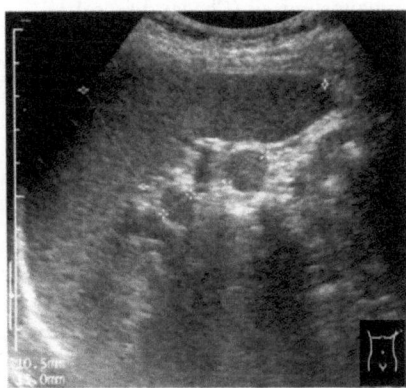

Fig. 2.18. Slightly enlarged spleen (pleuropneumonia). The pleural effusion enables the demonstration of the upper parts of the spleen. Normally the part left of the line would be covered by the acoustic shadow of the air-containing lung in the sinus

Fig. 2.19. Two small accessory spleens. The accessory spleens, close to the hilus of the spleen, should not be misinterpreted as enlarged lymph nodes

2.3.2.4
Pathologic Findings

Based on its function, the spleen is commonly involved in infectious and parasitic diseases (Table 2.2).

Two sonographic symptoms of inflammatory or infectious diseases can be seen, namely focal lesions and splenomegaly (Figs. 2.20–2.22).

An enlargement of the spleen can be seen in acute septicemic bacterial and virus infections, as well as in the chronic stage of such disorders. Splenomegaly is common in fungal infections and in protozoan diseases. The most common protozoan infections causing splenomegaly are malaria and leishmaniasis.

In areas where *Malaria falciparum* is endemic, the so-called "tropical splenomegaly" is very common. This may cause a differential diagnostic problem, since a splenomegaly (Fig. 2.20) demonstrated by ultrasound may exist independent from the acute situation.

Table 2.2. Major infectious (tropical) diseases affecting the spleen

Tuberculosis
Trypanosomiasis (Chagas disease)
Leishmaniasis (kala-azar)
Malaria (tropical splenomegaly syndrome)
Schistosomiasis
Hydatid disease
Clonorchiasis
Toxoplasmosis
Fungi, especially histoplasmosis
Porocephalosis
Malignant lymphomas
Hemoglobinopathies

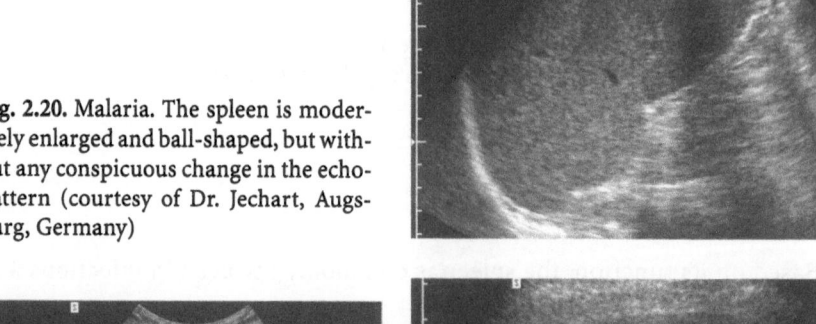

Fig. 2.20. Malaria. The spleen is moderately enlarged and ball-shaped, but without any conspicuous change in the echopattern (courtesy of Dr. Jechart, Augsburg, Germany)

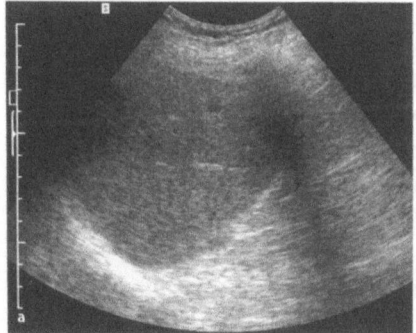 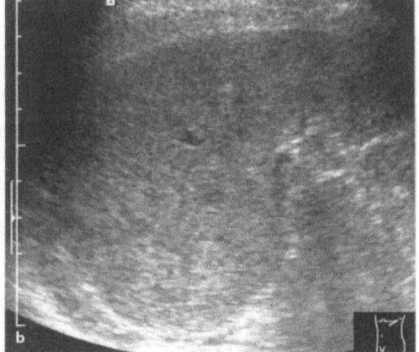

Fig. 2.21. a Enlarged spleen with a small pyogenic abscess (sepsis). **b** Enlarged spleen with small echo-poor focal lesions (malignant lymphoma)

Fig. 2.22. Spleen with old calcified tuber-culous nodes. (compare with Figs. 3.6, 3.16, and 3.63)

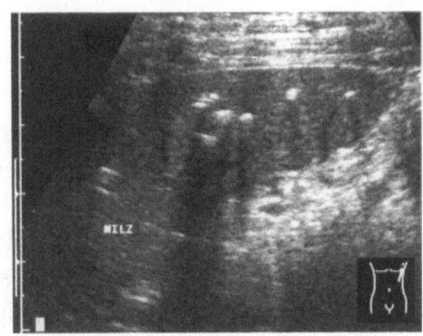

Tropical splenomegaly:
Idiopathic tropical splenomegaly is a clinical entity defined by a con-stellation of

- splenomegaly
- with or without liver involvement,
- elevated IGM levels,
- coagulopathy (secondarily),
- unclear etiology

Tropical splenomegaly in a more strict sense is seen in younger per-sons living in areas where malaria (*M. falciparum*) is endemic. The frequency of splenomegaly indicates the degree of infestation. The splenic index is defined as the number of cases of splenomegaly per 100 individuals examined (11–50 = hypoendemic, > 75 = hyperen-demic area).

Ultrasound is the most suitable method to demonstrate the splen-omegaly and for the follow-up controls under treatment.

The echo pattern of the sometimes enormously enlarged spleen is homogeneous. Ultrasound is useful to differentiate focal lesions caus-ing splenomegaly. Furthermore, the splenomegaly caused by portal hypertension can be differentiated (see Sects. 2.3.4 and 3.2.2).

On the other side, it must be taken in consideration that, in these ar-eas, a splenomegaly demonstrated by ultrasound in an acute situation may be independent from the actual problems of a patient.

2.3.2.5
Differential Diagnostic Aspects

In general splenomegaly is an nonspecific ultrasonic finding, since the echo pattern of the spleen is not altered in different ways by the different disorders (Fig. 2.21a,b).

Splenomegaly caused by hematological diseases cannot be differentiated, for the same reasons. Only in some cases of malignant lymphomas are focal lesions seen, additionally. Splenomegaly caused by portal hypertension may be distinguished based on the demonstration of collaterals or other symptoms of portal hypertension.

The mostly small accessory spleen should not be misinterpreted as an enlarged lymph node (Fig. 2.20).

> **Leishmania splenomegaly:**
> *Leishmania donovani* causes the visceral leishmaniasis, which is very common in many endemic parts of the world. Hepatosplenomegaly and increased skin pigmentation (kala-azar) occur.
>   Ultrasound is able to demonstrate the enlarged spleen with a uniform echo pattern as a nonspecific symptom.
>   Leishmania of the spleen or the liver causes an irregular echo pattern in some cases, thus mimicking a neoplastic disorder.

2.3.3
Lung and Pleura

2.3.3.1
Examination Technique

- Preparation not required
- Supine or sitting position, depending on the situation and the clinical inquiry
- Initially longitudinal scans, then oblique scans parallel to the ribs
- Lower parts of the pleural space can be demonstrated with subcostal scans through the liver or the spleen, respectively. The same technique is used to demonstrate pleural effusion.
- The anterior mediastinum is scanned on both sides of the sternum.

2.3.3.2
Normal Findings

– Normally only the chest wall, the diaphragm from subcostal area, and
  the heart can be seen. The ribs cause a line of strong echoes, but not in
  the cartilaginous part.
– Behind the chest wall or the diaphragm, a strong line of echoes reflected
  from the surface of the air-containing lung is seen.
– Echoes like those from a parenchymatous organ behind the diaphragm,
  demonstrated in subcostal scans, are mirror artifacts (see Fig. 3.22).

2.3.3.3
Indications

– pleural effusion
– pericardial effusion
– superficial lesions and masses of the lung (e.g., abscesses, hydatid cysts)
– processes in the anterior mediastinum
– (pneumonia)

2.3.3.4
Pathologic Findings

The ultrasonic examination of the organs of the chest is limited, because
ultrasound waves cannot penetrate through the ribs or through the air-
containing lung. Ultrasound is able only to demonstrate lesions and alterations of the pleura and at the surface of the air-containing lung. Naturally,
if the lung parenchyma is free of air, it can also be demonstrated.

Pleura
Most abnormalities of the pleura cause pleural effusion, which can easily be diagnosed by ultrasound as echo-free fluid (Fig. 2.23). Such an
echo-free serous pleural effusion is seen in tuberculosis (TB), but also in
noninflammatory diseases. Fluid caused by pleuritis contains more protein, which means fibrin. In these cases, fine echoes like threads can be
seen (Figs. 2.24, 2.28). In a later stage, the effusion becomes septate. Fine
echoes, sometimes sedimented, are typical for a purulent pleuritis, but
can also be seen in hemorrhagic effusions (Fig. 2.25). An empyema in the

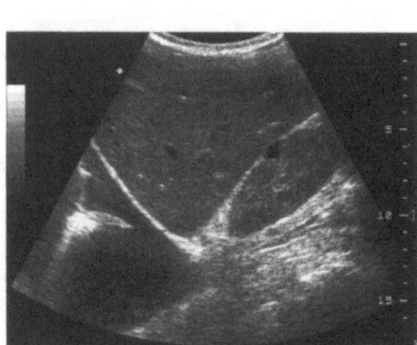 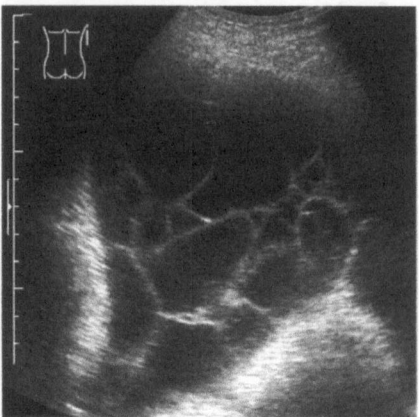

Fig. 2.23. Pleural effusion. Examination of the pleural space through the liver, with the patient in supine position. (Small cortical cyst in the right kidney)

Fig. 2.24. Exudative pleuritis. The net of fine echoes indicates the high content of fibrin (exudate)

pleural cavity sometimes shows a very complex pattern with strong echoes (gas, Figs. 2.7, 2.26). But, on the other hand, it cannot be excluded with safety, if there is only fluid without echoes.

It may be helpful to look to the surface of the lung, the diaphragm, and the chest wall (that is, the parietal and visceral pleura), or to the lung itself,

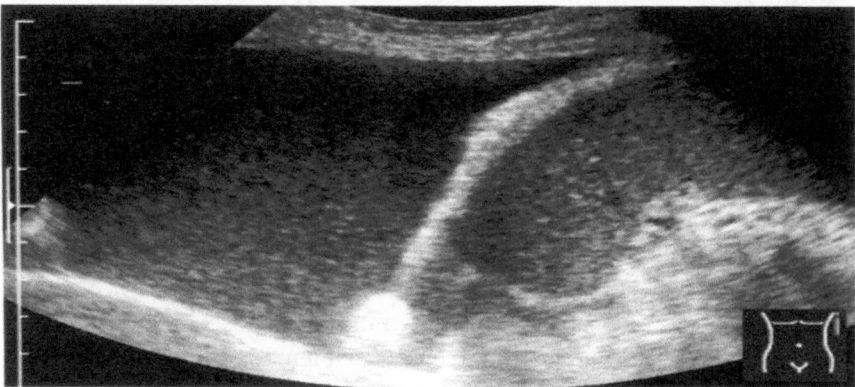

Fig. 2.25. Hemorrhagic pleural effusion. The fine echoes indicate sedimented particles in the fluid

Fig. 2.26. Encapsulated pleural empyema

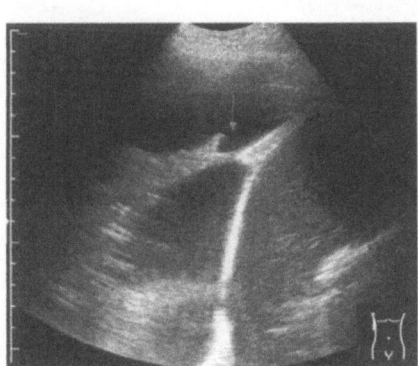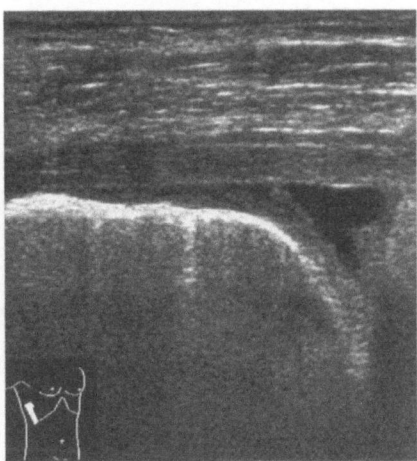

Fig. 2.27. Pleural effusion. The adhesion (*arrow*) indicates the beginning organization

Fig. 2.28. Pleuritis. Note the thickened pleura in front of the strong echoes caused by the air in the lung. The small line of fluid indicates the transition from the dry to the humid stage

to detect alterations such as an irregular surface or tumor tissue, and to find the reason.

In other cases, the ultrasonically guided puncture will be the method of choice to detect the nature of the effusion.

A circumscribed thickened pleura without fluid may be the late result of a pleuritis after organization of the effusion (Figs. 2.27, 2.28). It may be seen in neoplastic diseases of the pleura (metastases, mesothelioma) as well, but is not typical for an acute infectious disorder.

Lung

Parts of the lung tissue can be visualized, if the parenchyma is free of air. This is a typical finding in pneumonias, in which the alveoli are filled by inflammatory exudate. The bronchi are marked by strong echoes arising from the air (Figs. 2.29–2.31). In contrast to acute pneumonia, an atelectatic part of the lung (e.g., caused by a central tumor) is completely without air-echoes (because the bronchi are also free of air), and shows an echo pattern like that of a parenchymatous organ ("hepatization"). A similar picture is rarely seen in a scarring pneumonia ("carnefication"; Fig. 2.32).

Fig. 2.29. Pleuropneumonia. The visible part of the lung shows air (strong echoes) only in the bronchi, whereas the parenchyma is free of air

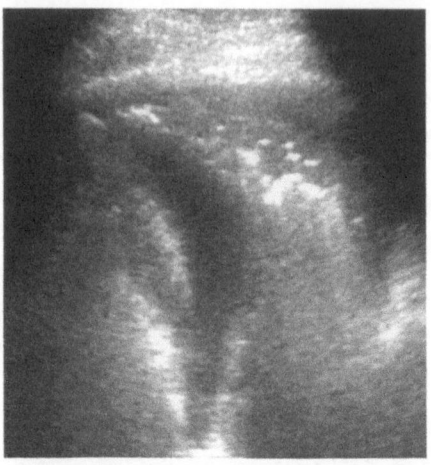

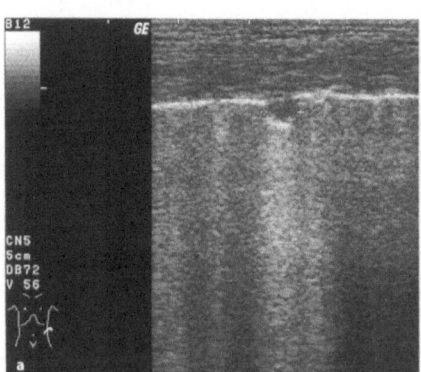

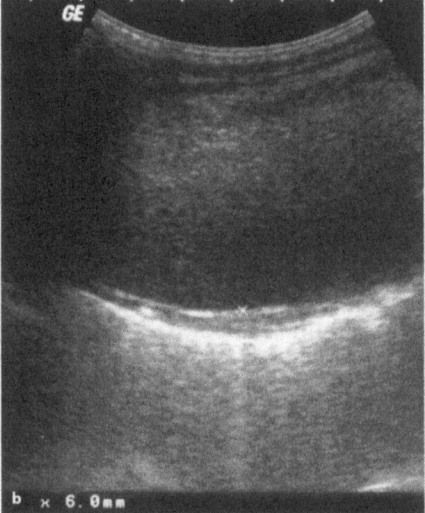

Fig. 2.30a,b. Tuberculosis of the lung. (a) Tuberculum at the surface of the lung. (Note the echoes arising on the surface of the normal lung and the artefacts caused by the air in the lung) (by courtesy of Dr. Gebhard Mathis, Hohenems, Austria) (b) Circumscribed tuberculous pleuritis (by courtesy of Dr. Gebhard Mathis, Hohenems, Austria)

Abscesses of the lung show the same variable, sometimes more echo-free (fluid), and sometimes very inhomogeneous echo pattern as empyemas of the pleura.

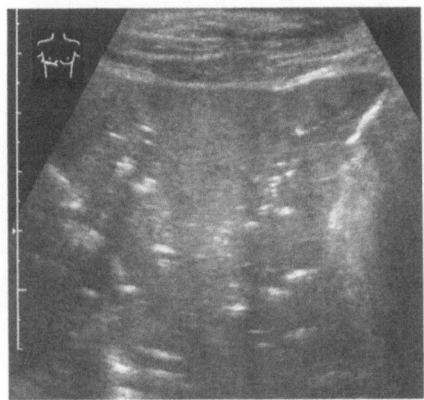 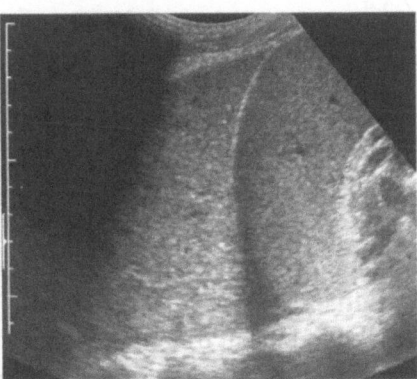

Fig. 2.31. Lobar pneumonia. The lung looks like a parenchymatous organ. Only a few strong echoes indicate some air bubbles in the larger bronchi

Fig. 2.32. Scarring of the lung (no resolution of a lobar pneumonia). The echo pattern of the lung looks like the echo pattern of the neighboring spleen. (The same sonographic finding is seen in atelectasis of a pulmonary lobe, caused by a central tumor)

If circumscribed lesions caused by parasites, e.g., hydatid cysts, are situated near the surface of the lung and not covered by air-filled parts of the lung, it is possible to detect them with ultrasound. Table 2.3 lists infectious diseases that infect the lung.

Table 2.3. Infectious (tropical) diseases affecting the lung

Tuberculosis (cosmopolitan)

Visceral leishmaniasis (bronchopneumonia)

Pneumocystis carinii infection (pneumonia, immunodeficient patients)

Schistosomiasis (bronchitis)

Hydatid disease

Lung trematode infection (cysts in the lung)

Strongyloidiasis (visceral larva migrans, causing transient eosinophilic pulmonary infiltrates, "tropical pulmonary eosinophilia")

Ancylostomiasis, syn.: uncinariasis (transient pulmonary infiltrates)

Toxocariasis (transient pulmonary infiltrates)

Ascaridiasis (pulmonary eosinophilic infiltrates, Löffler's syndrome)

2.3.4
Liver and Biliary Tract

2.3.4.1
Examination Technique

- Preparation not required, but the gallbladder is easier to demonstrate in a fasting patient.
- Supine position, left lateral decubitus if necessary
- Initially longitudinal scans, starting left to the midline, demonstrating the left lobe in front of the aorta. Systematic scans to the left margin of the liver and then to the right flank in deep inspiration
- Additionally, oblique subcostal and–if needed–intercostal scans parallel to the ribs, especially to demonstrate the vessels. Finally, transverse or oblique scans through the hilus to demonstrate the portal vein and the common bile duct
- Measurements: longitudinal diameter right mid-clavicular line (right of the gall bladder). Thickness of the left lobe in front of the aorta. Diameter of the portal vein.
- The examination must include the gallbladder, bile ducts, and the spleen.
- For the examination of the common bile duct, 45° left lateral decubitus is most satisfactory.

2.3.4.2
Normal Findings

- Vertical diameter in the right MCL < 12 cm, but wide variations depending on the shape of the liver. Thickness of the left lobe < 6 cm, measured in front of the aorta.
- Surface smooth. Inferior edge is wedge-shaped, the angle depending on the habitus.
- The echo pattern is uniform. The density is similar to that of the parenchyma of the kidney (Fig. 2.33a–c).
- The intrahepatic vessels and ducts are well delineated, especially the portal vein branches and the hepatic veins. The branches of the portal vein show strong echoes from the wall.
- The diameter of the portal vein less than 12 mm, the cross-section should be oval and the caliber should vary depending on breathing. Blood flow hepatopetal. Mean flow velocity 15–22 cm/s (variable data in the literature).

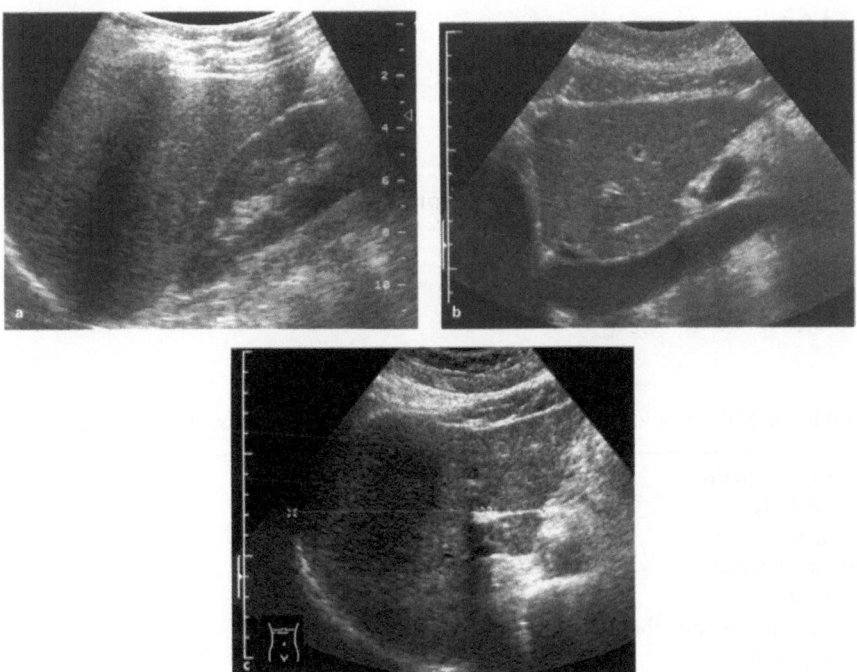

Fig. 2.33a–c. Liver, normal findings. Longitudinal scan right lobe (**a**) and left lobe in front of the caval vein (**b**), Transverse scan (**c**) with measurement of the right lobe and the caudate lobe

- Hepatic artery: diameter 4–10 mm, mean flow velocity (Vmean) 20–40 cm/s, RI 0.6–0.7.
- Hepatic veins: diameter < 10 mm (measured 1 cm distal to the vena cava).Triphasic flow (in 75%), depending on the cardiac cycle
- The gall bladder is visualized at the edge of the liver as an oval echo-free organ with a thin wall (< 3 mm if not contracted). The size and the shape are variable. The transverse diameter should be less than 4 cm.
- The common bile duct is visualized in front of the portal vein and the right branch of the hepatic artery, with a diameter less than 8 mm.

2.3.4.3
Indications

– Systemic inflammatory diseases
– Fever
– Palpable masses in the upper abdomen
– Virus hepatitis
– Chronic liver disorders
– Protozoan diseases (Table 2.4)

Table 2.4. Major tropical diseases affecting the liver and biliary tract

Virus – hepatitis
Amebiasis
Schistosomiasis
Hydatid disease
Ascariasis
Clonorchiasis and other liver fluke diseases
Toxoplasmosis
Kala-azar
Chagas disease
Fungal diseases, especially histoplasmosis
Porocephalosis
Kwashiorkor

2.3.4.4
Pathologic Findings

The liver as a central metabolic organ can be affected by a large number of different diseases ranging from inborn metabolic disorders to neoplastic diseases. Not least, a remarkable number of infectious organisms may cause diseases of the liver, especially viruses and parasites. Whereas parasites and pyogenic bacteria cause mainly larger focal alterations and lesions, virus infections cause diffuse microscopic alterations. The first are detected as focal lesions by ultrasound, whereas in the latter diseases, only an enlargement of the liver can be seen without any specific change of the echo pattern (see Chap. 3, Sect. 3.2.2).

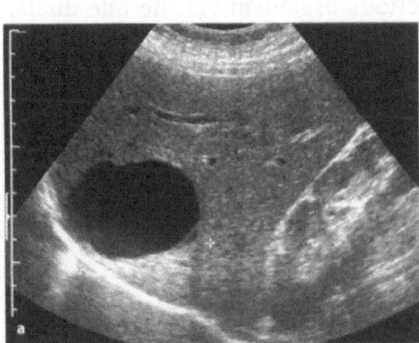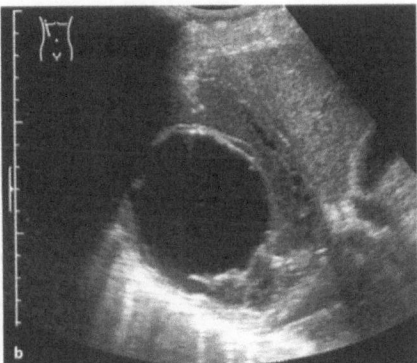

Fig. 2.34a,b. Cystic lesions in the liver. The oval, smooth and echo-free lesion, 60 mm in size (**a**), corresponds to a dysontogenetic cyst. However, a hydatid cyst (type I Gharbi classification; see Sect. 3.3.7.1) must be considered in differential diagnosis. The second lesion (**b**) shows an atypical broad wall, which is never seen in a harmless dysontogenetic cyst: hydatid cyst

The great variety of liver diseases presents a special challenge for ultrasound, as for each other diagnostic method. Focal lesions such as abscesses or parasitic lesions must be differentiated from benign or malignant neoplastic processes or inborn cystic lesions. The echo pattern of a hydatid cyst stage I looks like a congenital cyst, for example. But a thickened wall is always nontypical for a congenital cyst (Fig. 2.34a,b).

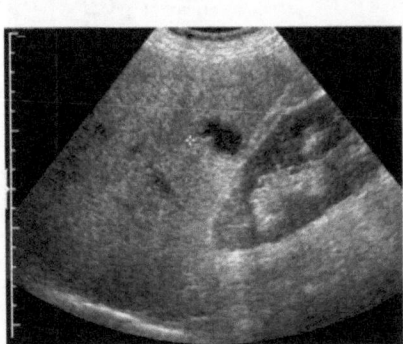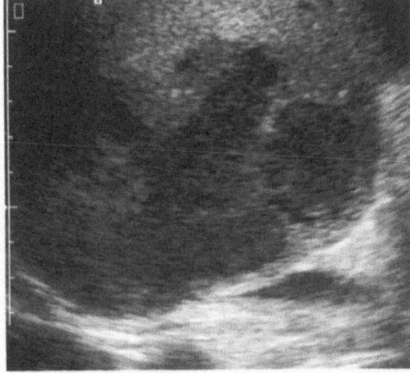

Fig. 2.35. Small (20-mm) pyogenic hepatic abscess. The abscess is nearly echo-free (type 1) and shows acoustic enhancement behind

Fig. 2.36. Amoebic abscess in the liver. The abscess, situated dorsally in the right hepatic lobe, shows an echo-poor pattern (type 2) and a irregular contour (courtesy of Dr. Jechart, Augsburg, Germany)

Pyogenic abscesses caused by infectious organism via the bile ducts, the portal vein, the hepatic artery, or spreading from a neighboring organ or a wound show extremely variable features ranging from echo-free fluid collections, imitating a cyst, to inhomogeneous lesions with strong echoes, indicating gas bubbles (Figs. 2.35–2.37). The common "solid" echo-poor pattern (tumor-like pattern) must be differentiated from a true neoplastic lesion. Compared to malignant lesions, hepatic abscesses are char-

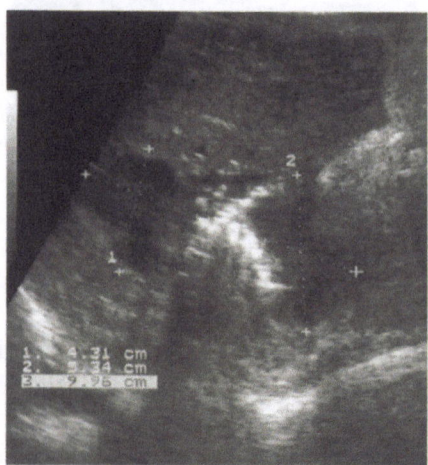

Fig. 2.37. Pyogenic hepatic abscess. Note the strong echoes indicating gas.

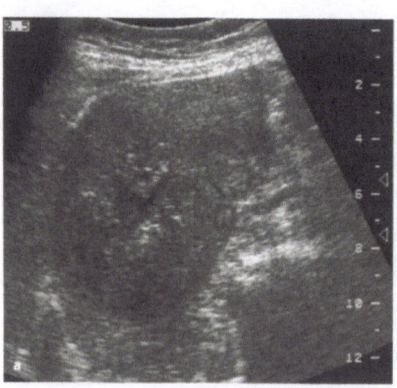

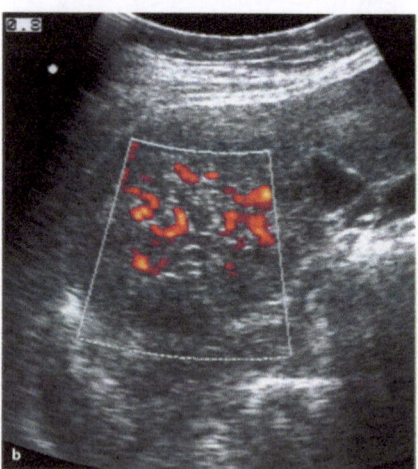

Fig. 2.38a,b. Hepatocellular carcinoma. The tumor shows an inhomogeneous pattern (**a**) similar to an (older) abscess, but with power Doppler, the typical hypervascularity can be seen (**b**)

acterized by a sharp contour and a more irregular "coalescent" shape (Fig. 2.38a).

Doppler examination may be necessary to differentiate between abscesses and hypervascular tumors based on Doppler signals from inside the lesion (Fig. 2.38b); but to distinguish between abscesses and hypovascular malignant tumors, mainly metastases, the use of contrast agents seems to be useful. With this technique the lack of internal enhancement is typical for hepatic abscesses in opposite to the malignant lesions (see Fig. 2.35a–c). On the other hand the hypervascular periphery, typical for pyogenic abscesses, is missed in amoebic abscesses.

A diffuse enlargement of the liver may be caused by a virus hepatitis as well as by a metabolic disorder or chronic intoxication, especially by alcohol.

Insofar as chronic diseases of the liver are common in many areas of the world, in endemic areas for virus hepatitis as well as in areas with alcohol abuse, clinicians should always consider the possibility of a combination of these diseases. Besides a parasitic disease such as a schistosomiasis, there may exist a liver cirrhosis independent from the parasitic disease and caused by a former hepatitis B infection or by alcoholism.

Jaundice is a typical symptom of liver diseases, but also may be caused by biliary obstruction. The differentiation between hepatic and obstructive jaundice needs just one "ultrasonic" view to the bile ducts, which are dilated in obstructive jaundice (Figs. 2.39, 2.40). The reason may be a tumor of the bile ducts or of the pancreas, or a stone. But it can be also

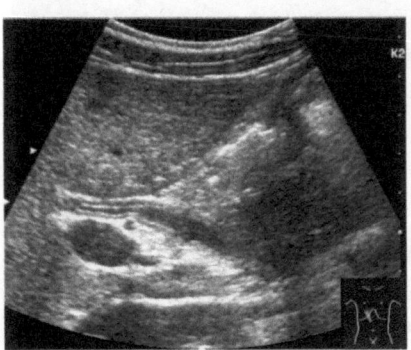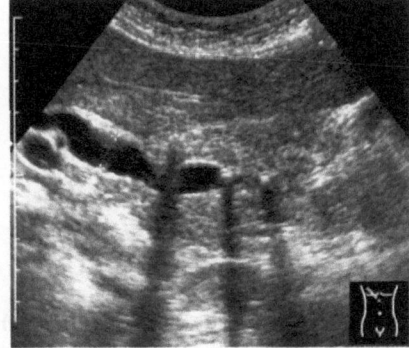

Fig. 2.39. Cholangitis. The common bile duct is not dilated, but shows a thickened wall

Fig. 2.40. Dilated common bile duct. Strong echoes with acoustic shadows indicate stones in the duct

a complication of a parasitic disease of the liver, e.g., of echinococcosis (see Chap. 3, Sect. 3.3.7).

The thickened wall of the bile ducts is seen in acute cholangitis (Fig. 2.39), but also in various parasitic diseases (see Chap. 3, Sects. 3.2.1, 3.3.5, 3.3.6) and in sclerosing cholangitis.

The ultrasonic symptom of an acute inflammation of the gall bladder (acute cholecystitis) seems to be the thickened wall (> 3 mm) at first sight (Figs. 2.41, 2.42). However, an increased thickness of the gall bladder wall is seen in a number of nonbiliary disorders as well. The underlying edema of the wall in these cases is caused by portal hypertension, by low osmotic pressure (hypoproteinemia) or by augmented extravascular fluid volume. A thickened wall can be demonstrated regularly in the late stage of liver cirrhosis (Fig. 2.43), in congestive heart disease with ascites, and in disorders causing hypoalbuminemia. Furthermore, a thickened wall of the gall bladder may be seen in schistosomiasis malaria falciparum, in patients with amoebic liver abscesses, and in various viral diseases such as in infectious mononucleosis, virus hepatitis, Dengue fever, and AIDS (see Chap. 3, Sect. 3.2 and 3.3.6).

Typical for the noninflammatory thickened wall are the symptoms of the underlying disorders, ascites or an edema around the gall bladder. Characteristic of an acute cholecystitis are the pain, provoked by transducer

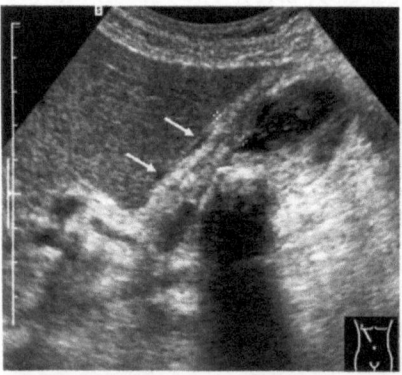 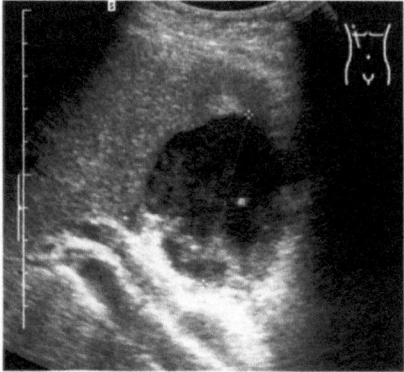

Fig. 2.41. Acute cholecystitis. The wall of the gall bladder is thickened (9 mm) and shows an irregular pattern. In the lumen, there are fine echoes and strong echoes with acoustic shadows indicating stones. The *arrows* mark a thin line of pericholecystic fluid (compare with Fig. 3.11)

Fig. 2.42. Empyema of the gall bladder. Note the echoes within the lumen. Behind the gall bladder, the common bile duct and the portal vein are seen

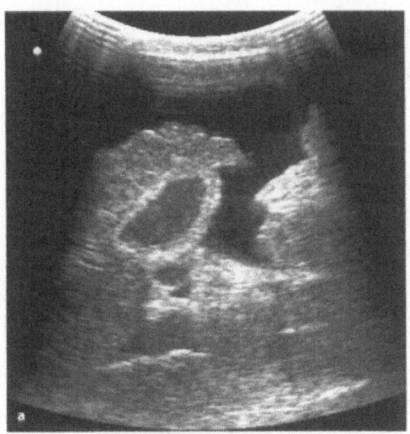
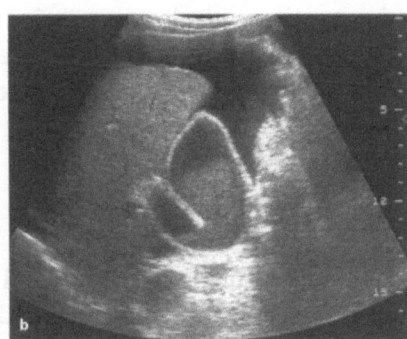

Fig. 2.43a,b. Differential diagnosis of ascites. The thickened wall of the gall bladder indicates benign serous ascites; the coarse surface of the liver identifies cirrhosis as the underlying disease (**a**). The normal wall of the gall bladder is very suspicious of a malignant ascites (**b**). Note the fine sedimented echoes in the gall bladder, so-called sludge

pressure (so-called "positive Murphy's sign") and the hyperemia demonstrated with color-Doppler. Stones are common in acute cholecystitis, but the lack of stones does not exclude an acute inflammation. In empyemas, weak irregular echoes may be seen in the lumen. However, this finding is not specific, but may be seen as "sludge" in fasting patients (Figs. 2.42, 2.43b).

Ascites caused by a malignant disease does not induce edema of the gall bladder wall. The thickened wall demonstrated in patients with ascites therefore indicates a benign disease (Fig. 2.43a,b).

2.3.5
Gastrointestinal Tract

2.3.5.1
Examination Technique

- High-frequency transducer (about 5 MHz) should be used.
- For the examination of the stomach, the water contrast method gives the best results (300–500 ml fluid without gas, eventually stopping the peristalsis with Buscopan). No preparation for the lower digestive tract necessary

- Supine position, right or left decubitus additionally
- Longitudinal and transverse scans of the area of interest, always starting in a section with clear anatomic conditions (liver, kidneys, aorta, etc)
- Slight pressure with the transducer improves the results by pressing the bowels' contents (air) out of the region of interest.

2.3.5.2
Normal Findings

The lower part of the esophagus and the cardia can be seen mostly behind the left liver lobe as a tubular formation. In the same way, the lower part of the stomach can be demonstrated. Only if the stomach is filled with fluid (water contrast method), the wall of all parts can be seen with a diameter of less than 4 mm. With a high-quality transducer, the different layers can be distinguished (Fig. 2.44a–c).

The visibility of the lower intestinal tract depends on its contents and on the quality of the equipment as well. With suitable transducers, all sections of the colon can be demonstrated with a wall not more than 3 mm thick (Fig. 2.45).

2.3.5.3
Indications

- pain in the abdomen
- suspicion on bowel obstruction
- palpable masses in the abdomen
- diarrhea lasting more than usual

2.3.5.4
Pathologic Findings

Segments of the gastrointestinal tract (GI) affected by an infectious organism (Table 2.5) usually react with a swelling of the mucosa and submucosa in the acute phase, a focal necrosis of the mucosa, which means ulceration and a malfunction. The malfunction of the small and large bowel causes the leading symptom of the (lower) GI tract, diarrhea.

Additionally, there may be a regional lymphadenitis and the appearance of ascites. As typical complications of these disorders, paralytic or

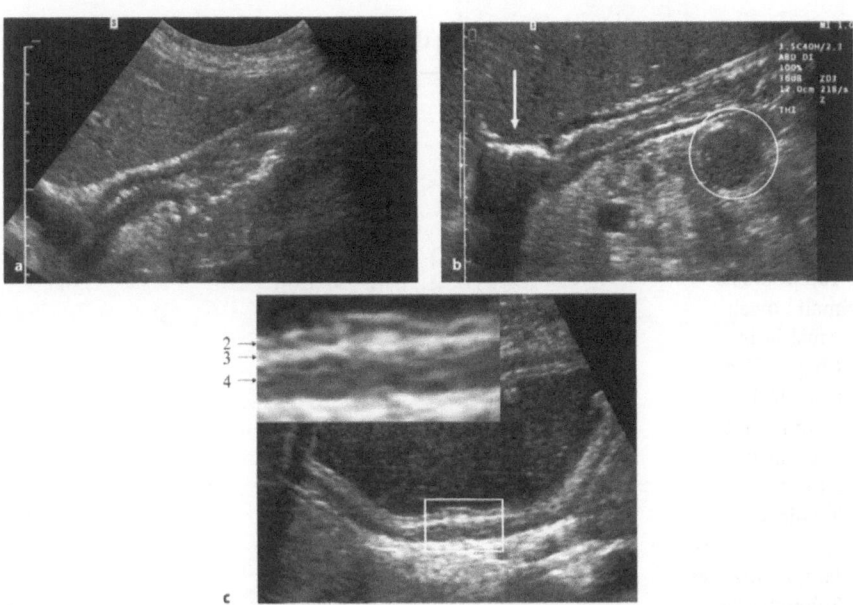

Fig. 2.44a–c. Stomach, normal findings. Entrance of the stomach (cardia) and the upper part of the body behind the left hepatic lobe (**a**). Distal part of the stomach behind the liver. The different layers of the wall are seen. The *arrow* marks air in the duodenal bulb. Behind the antrum, parts of the pancreas. The echo-poor figure (O) corresponds to the distal part of the duodenum (**b**). The technique of "water contrast" is the best method for the examination of the stomach: the wall of the body is well demonstrated, even with 3.5 MHz. The arrows in the detail mark the anatomic layers: 2, echo-poor, = mucosa, 3, echo-rich, = submucosa and 4, echo-poor, = muscle layer, whereas the first echo-rich line and the fifth echo-rich line are caused by the interface between the wall and the lumen and the surrounding tissue, respectively (**c**)

Fig. 2.45. Small bowel loops, normal find-ing

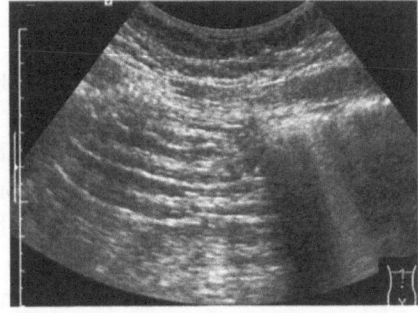

Table 2.5. Major tropical diseases affecting the gastrointestinal tract

Stomach:
  Schistosomiasis
  Ascariasis
  Anisakiasis
  Strongyloidiasis
  Fungal diseases (candidiasis)
  Tuberculosis
Small bowel:
  Amebiasis
  Chagas disease
  Giardiasis
  Strongyloidiasis
  Ascariasis
  Anisakiasis
  Taeniasis
  Hookworm disease
  Fungal diseases
  Tuberculosis
  Tropical sprue
Colon and rectum:
  Amebiasis
  Schistosomiasis
  Chagas disease
  Ascariasis
  Strongyloidiasis
  Trichiuriasis
  Helminthoma
  Fungal diseases, especially actinomycosis

mechanical bowel obstruction, fistulas (amebiasis), or a perforation may occur.

With ultrasound, the circumscribed or segmental thickening of the gastric or bowel wall can be demonstrated in general as a nonspecific symptom of these disorders. Using high-resolution equipment, the various layers of the thickened wall can be differentiated. This may be helpful in some situations, since benign diseases do not involve the muscle layer.

Some of the ulcers of the stomach or the duodenum can be seen, if a high-resolution instrument and the water contrast technique are used, but the exclusion of such a lesion is not possible (Figs. 2.46–2.51).

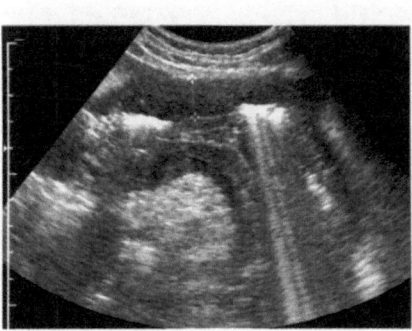 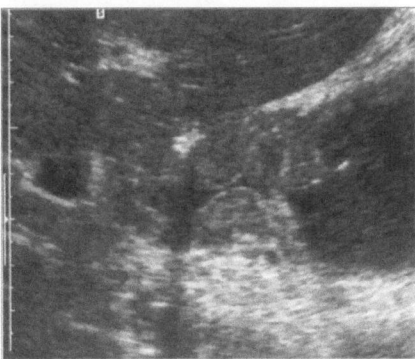

Fig. 2.46. Thickened gastric wall (14 mm). In this case the thickening was caused by severe acute bacterial gastritis

Fig. 2.47. Duodenal ulcer. The wall of the duodenal wall is swollen. A strong echo (air) in the anterior part marks the deep ulcer

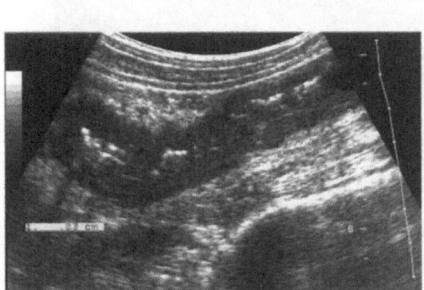 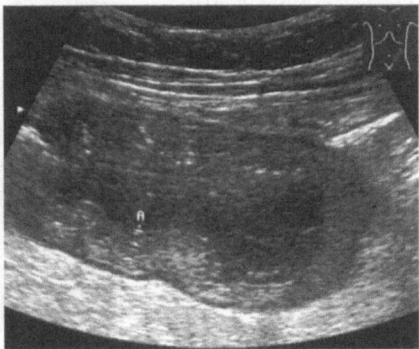

Fig. 2.48. Ulcerative colitis, acute stage. Descending colon with a thickened, echo-poor wall; the narrowed lumen marked by some strong echoes (gas bubbles)

Fig. 2.49. Acute pseudomembranous colitis (*Clostridium difficile*). The oblique scan through a segment of the colon shows an edematous thickened wall (11 mm). The different layers are still distinguishable; the edema includes especially the submucosal layer

Ascites is easy to detect, even very small amounts. Enlarged lymph nodes also can be demonstrated, for example, in the ileocecal region (see Fig. 2.17).

The hyperperistalsis of the bowel can be seen with real-time ultrasound, as can the bowel obstruction. Whereas the fluid-filled intestinal loops are not dilated in simple diarrhea, the dilatation combined with hyperperistalsis is typical of the spastic type of obstruction (Fig. 2.52). In paralytic bowel

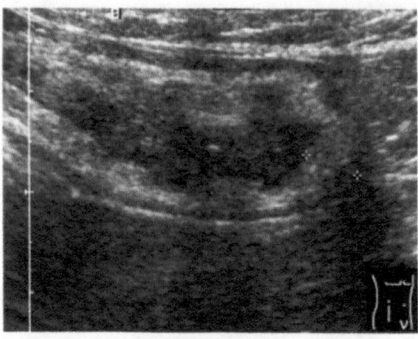 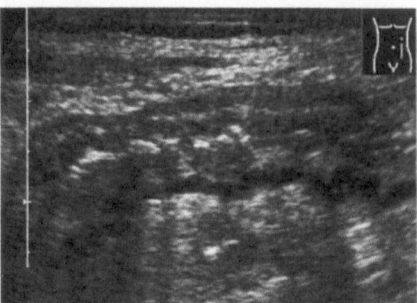

Fig. 2.50. Amoebic colitis (+ – + 9 mm)

Fig. 2.51. Malignant lymphoma of the colon. The different layers are still distinguishable. The image is not different from the images of inflammatory colitis (compare with Fig. 2.50)

Fig. 2.52. Bowel obstruction

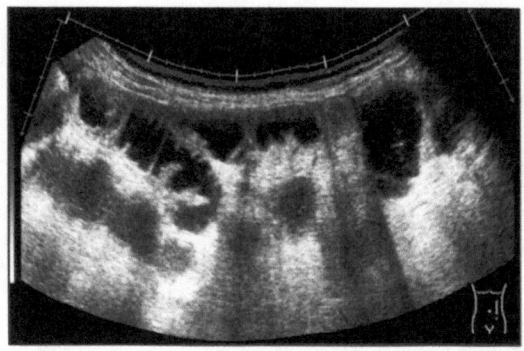

obstruction, only a slow or even no movement of the dilated loops is seen. In this case, one can only see movement through breathing or pulsation, whereas the content of the bowel is sedimented (Fig. 2.53). Strong echoes within the wall – pneumatosis intestinalis – is more typical of ischemic colitis, but may be demonstrated in severe infectious colitis as a symptom of poor prognosis (Fig. 2.54a,b). Fistulas are demonstrated as echo-poor structures, but in reality, the echo-poor areas correspond to the inflammation around the fistulas, whereas the fistula itself is marked by some stronger echoes (Fig. 2.55).

Free perforations are diagnosed by the demonstration of free air in the abdomen. In order to avoid misinterpretations, the air bubbles should be demonstrated in front of the right liver lobe, the highest point of the

Fig. 2.53. Paralytic bowel obstruction. Between the dilated small bowel loops, ascites. (No peristalsis is seen in real time)

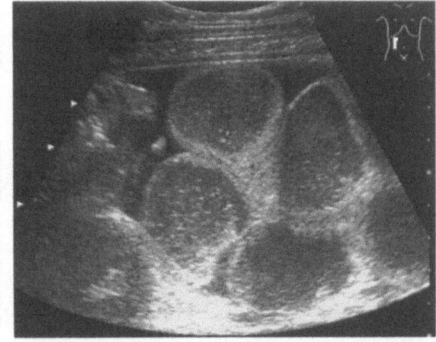

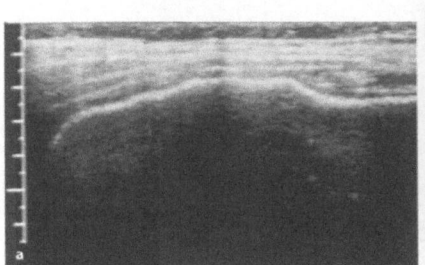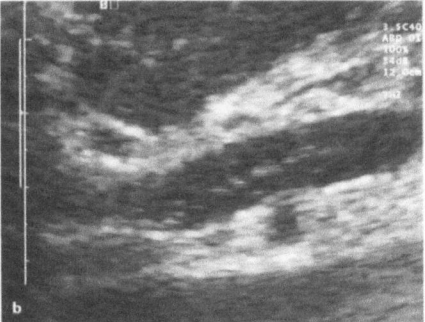

Fig. 2.54a,b. Pneumatosis intestinalis. Gas in the anterior wall of the transverse colon, which causes an acoustic shadow behind and reverberation artifacts (**a**). Gas bubbles in the portal vein (**b**)

abdomen if the patient has a slight oblique position, because there are normally no air-containing structures (Fig. 2.56a,b).

Again it must be mentioned that all of these ultrasonic findings are not pathognomonic for certain (infectious or parasitic) diseases. The same findings, a focal or segmental thickening of the wall, may be seen in non-infectious inflammatory diseases (e.g., Crohn's disease) and even malignant diseases, especially lymphomas (Fig. 2.51), as well. Even the use of Doppler techniques, e.g., to demonstrate the hyperemia of the wall affected, does not allow a differential diagnosis, with the exception of the ischemic colitis.

Fig. 2.55. Inflammatory tumor. Conglomerate of inflamed mesentery, involved sections of the bowel, fluid, and short fistulas (*arrow*)

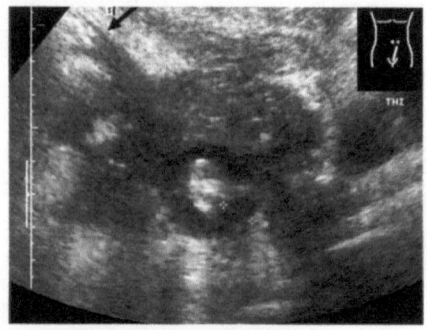

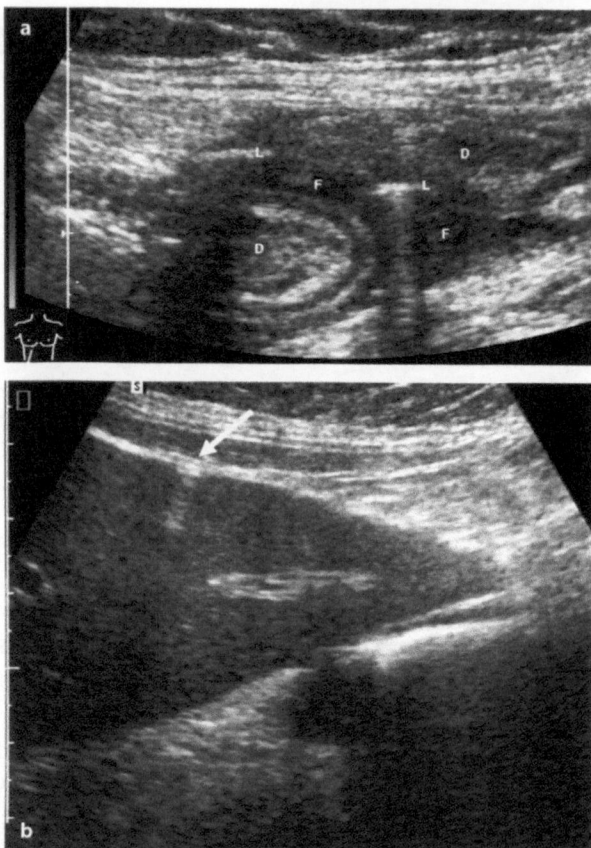

Fig. 2.56a,b. Free perforation. Air bubble (L) in the fluid (F) between inflamed bowel loops (D) (**a**). Air bubble, causing characteristic artifacts, in front of the right hepatic lobe (*arrow*). (**b**) This finding proves the perforation

2.3.6
Kidney

2.3.6.1
Examination Technique

- Preparation not required
- Supine or left and right decubitus. Alternatively prone position
- Longitudinal scans and transverse scans including the vessels
- Measurement of the length and the diameter of the parenchyma

2.3.6.2
Normal Findings

- Ovoid shape with a diameter of > 10 cm. Thickness of the parenchyma > 11 mm. The pyramids are more echo-poor than the cortex (good contrast in children, less in elderly persons).
- The bright echoes in the center or hilus, respectively, correspond to the wall of the renal pelvis, the large vessels, and fatty tissue. Normally no fluid is seen in the pelvis.
- The fat capsule around the kidney shows a more echo-rich, "coarse grained" pattern causing a strong contrast to the cortex. The thickness of this fat capsule varies widely. In lean persons, only a thin line of bright echoes may be seen (Fig. 2.57a,b).

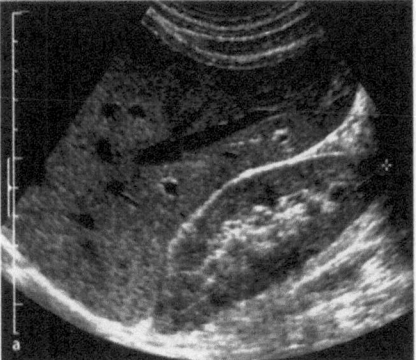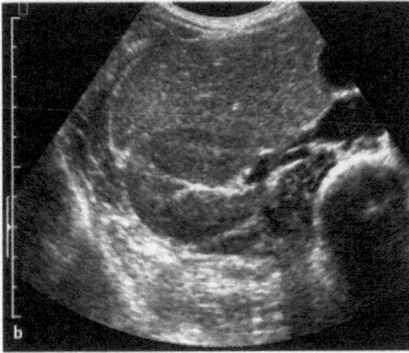

Fig. 2.57a,b. Right kidney, normal findings. Longitudinal scan shows the long axis of the kidney behind the right hepatic lobe (**a**). Transverse scan shows the renal vessels in front of the muscles and the spine. On the side, the caval vein and a part of the gall-bladder (**b**)

- Renal artery: diameter 5–8 mm, Vmax 60–180 cm/s, RI 0.6–0.7. Difference between right and left kidney < 10%.

2.3.6.3
Indications

- pain in the flank
- fever
- acute or chronic renal failure
- in connection with protozoan diseases
- tuberculosis

2.3.6.4
Pathologic Findings

Bacterial infections of the urinary tract are very common. The pathogenic organisms may reach the kidneys ascending from the lower tract (usually) or seldom with the blood. Ascending infections are common, especially in females. They are generally promoted by obstructions or reflux.

In acute pyelonephritis, a slight enlargement of the kidney(s) can be demonstrated as a nonspecific sign (Fig. 2.58). In the cortex, small abscesses can be seen, as echo-poor or echo-free lesions. If the treatment is not adequate, larger abscesses will develop, and they will spread to the perirenal area. In those cases, an echo-poor area extending from the kidney can be seen. The shape of the lesion may be irregular. If there are gas bubbles, intensive (bright) echoes, sometimes causing a shadow, are seen.

A dilated renal pelvis is seen, especially if obstruction is present as a cofactor of the inflammatory disease. The fluid within the pelvis may be

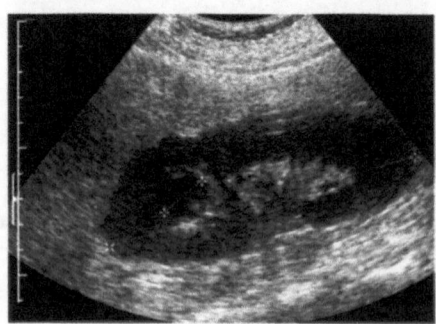

Fig. 2.58. Acute pyelonephritis. The right kidney shows an echo-poor pattern and is enlarged (13 cm). One calix is dilated

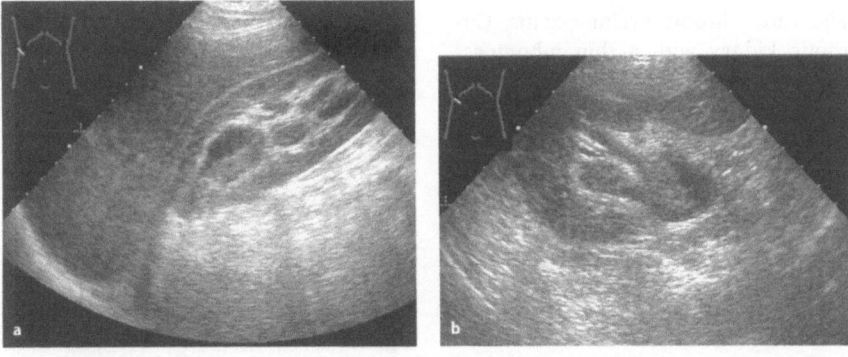

Fig. 2.59a,b. Purulent acute pyelonephritis. The pelvis is dilated, and the fluid shows "sedimented" echoes (pus)

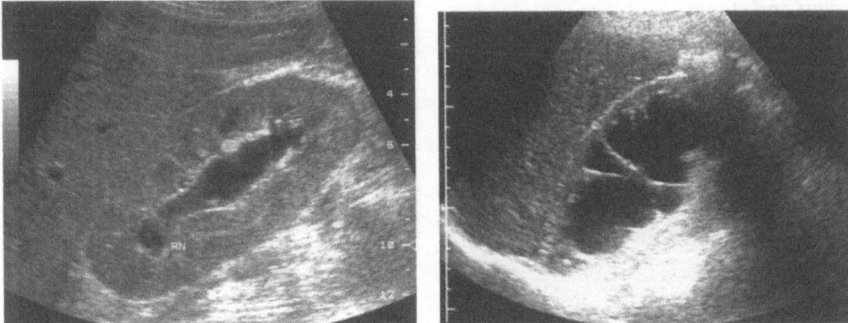

Fig. 2.60. Acute renal outflow obstruction. The parenchyma is somewhat swollen due to edema

Fig. 2.61. Hydronephrosis. Compared to acute stasis (Fig. 2.60), the parenchyma of the kidney is thin, which indicates a chronic obstruction

echo-free, but sometimes few (sedimented) echoes can be seen within the fluid (Figs. 2.59a,b–2.61).

In the chronic stage of pyelonephritis, the kidney parenchyma becomes smaller, leading to a general reduction of kidney size at the end. The echo pattern of the parenchyma becomes irregular and more echo-dense. Scars are seen as bright areas in the cortex, causing a retraction of the surface. The shape becomes especially irregular if only a part of the kidney is shrunken (Fig. 2.62).

Xanthogranulomatous pyelonephritis is a special variant of chronic pyelonephritis, mostly in combination with stones. Usually only one kidney is affected. The kidney is enlarged, the pelvis dilated, and stones are seen as strong echoes with shadows (Fig. 2.63).

Fig. 2.62. Chronic pyelonephritis. Cirrhotic kidney with a thin inhomogeneous parenchyma

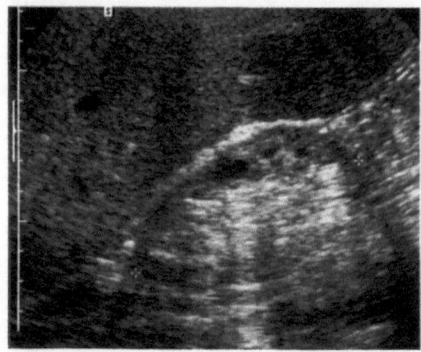

Fig. 2.63. Xanthogranulomatous pyelonephritis. Right kidney shows dilated pelvis and stones

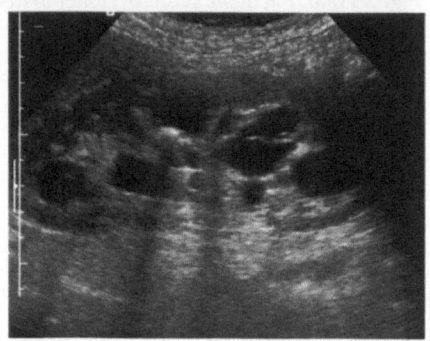

The rare hematogenic infections cause abscesses, often without connection to the renal pelvis.

2.3.6.5
Differential Diagnosis (Table 2.6)

Table 2.6. Major tropical diseases affecting the kidneys

Tuberculosis
Hydatid disease
Schistosomiasis

The enlargement of the kidney in the acute stage of an infectious disease is a nonspecific reaction, but can be seen in all the other acute disorders affecting the kidneys such as toxic damage or noninfectious inflammatory diseases.

Tuberculosis of the kidneys is the most common extrapulmonary manifestation of this disease.

Echo-poor abscesses or dilated calices can be demonstrated by ultrasound in the same way as in other bacterial infections (Fig. 2.64; see Chap. 3, Sect. 3.1.).

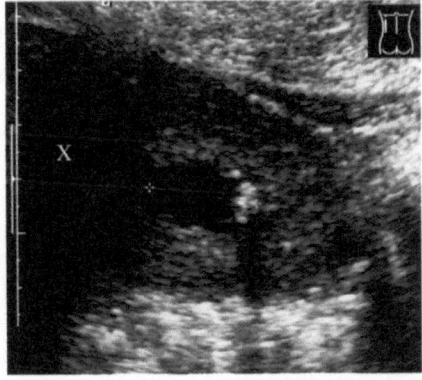

Fig. 2.64. Renal tuberculosis. Left kidney shows a dilated calix (21 mm) with calcification. (X = shadow of a rib)

Furthermore, tumors and lymphomas of the kidney must be taken into account if an echo-poor lesion is seen. The differentiation based on grayscale technique may be difficult in some cases. However, neoplasms can

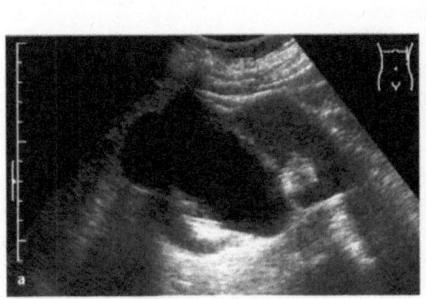
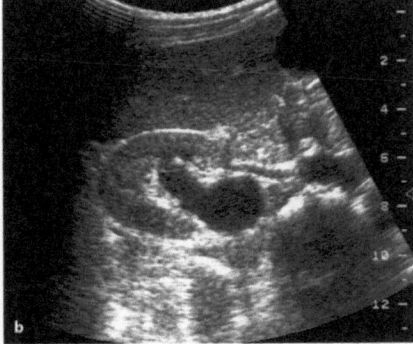

Fig. 2.65a,b. Differential diagnosis of renal cyst. Cyst of the right kidney. Central situated renal cysts may imitate hydronephrosis, especially in the longitudinal scan (a). Cross-section clearly shows (in another case) a dilated renal pelvis (b). Anterior to the dilated pelvis, the renal artery is seen

be distinguished from abscesses on grounds of Doppler signals arising within the lesion, if the technique is available. An alternative procedure is ultrasonically guided fine-needle puncture.

Even simple renal cysts may cause differential diagnostic problems, especially if the clinical background is not noticed. These cysts are common, especially in elderly persons. The ultrasonic findings (echo-free, smooth outline, seldom septate) are the same as in hydatid cysts of stage I or II (see Chap. 3, Sect. 3.3.7).

A number of centrally situated cysts can imitate the ultrasonic picture of hydronephrosis, especially in the longitudinal scan. The differentiation should be possible with the transverse scan additionally (Fig. 2.65a,b).

CHAPTER 3

Ultrasound Diagnosis of Special Infectious and Parasitic Diseases

3.1
Bacterial Infections

3.1.1
Ultrasound in Extrapulmonary Tuberculosis
(by Mohamed Salah Kechaou, Sana Mezghani, Zeineb Mnif, Jamel Mnif)

3.1.1.1
Introduction

Pulmonary involvement is the most frequent tuberculosis location. If ultrasonography is not adapted to study this location as a matter of routine, it can still be used as a technique for exploration of the other abdomino-pelvic locations and soft tissues. It represents a real extension of the palpating hand. This technique is safe, cheap, and repetitive.

The extrapulmonary tuberculosis lesions (e.g., nodes, lymph nodes, abscess) are well studied by ultrasonography.

The recent advances in ultrasound technology (high-frequency probes, harmonic imaging, contrast agent) have made the investigation of the bowel loops highly practicable.

3.1.1.2
Abdominal Tuberculosis

Abdominal tuberculosis may affect the gastro-intestinal tract, the peritoneum, the lymph nodes, and the solid viscera. This disease may affect these organs separately, but the involvement of multiple viscera is highly suggestive of the diagnosis.

Ultrasound is usually performed initially. Its advantage is that it allows the investigation of all abdominal and pelvic organs at the same time.

Ultrasound findings are not specific, but some features can suggest tuberculosis diagnosis, especially in patients at risk.

Fine-needle aspiration biopsy guided by ultrasound is very helpful for obtaining cytological and histopathological confirmation of the diagnosis.

Ultrasound also permits the follow-up of patients under chemotherapy.

3.1.1.3
Gastrointestinal Tract

The ileocecal region is the most common area of involvement in the gastrointestinal tract, due to the abundance of lymphoid tissue.

Ultrasonography may show uniform and circumferential wall thickening of the cecum and terminal ileum associated with adjacent mesenteric lymphadenopathy (Fig. 3.1). Occasionally, ulceration is visible.

The involvement of the ileum and cecum may cause this area to be retracted into the subhepatic region, producing the "pseudo-kidney" sign.

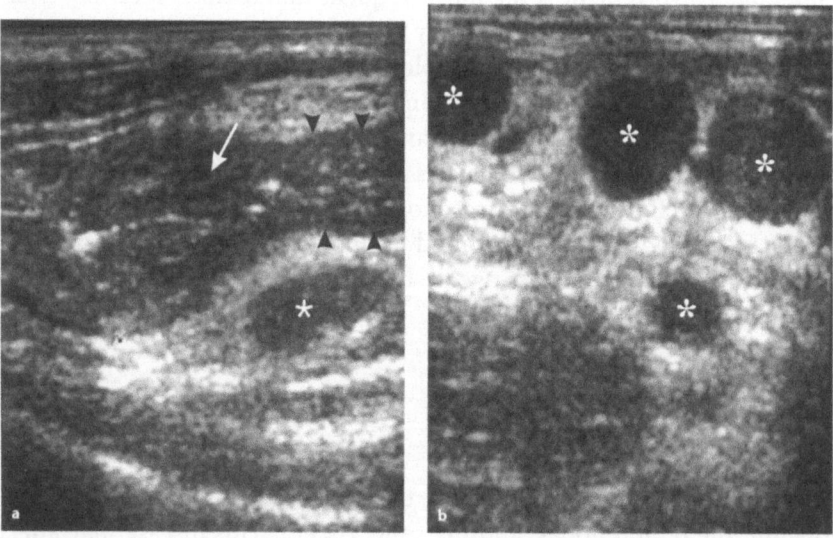

Fig. 3.1a,b. Ileocecal tuberculosis. Ultrasound (US) images of the right lower quadrant show a wall thickening of terminal ileum (*arrowheads*) and thickening of the ileocecal valve (*arrow*) (**a**) with regional hypoechoic lymph nodes (*asterisk*, **b**)

3.1.1.4
Peritoneal Tuberculosis

Tuberculosis in peritoneal location is one of the most common extrapulmonary manifestations.

Three types of tuberculosis in this location have been described: they are a "wet" type with free or loculated fluid, a "dry" type with caseous nodules and adhesions, and a fibrotic-fixed type with mass formation consisting of omentum and loops of intestine or mesentery, sometimes with ascites (Fig. 3.2).

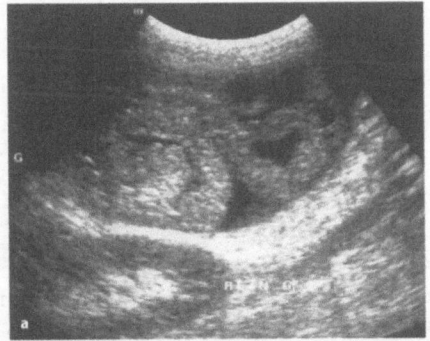

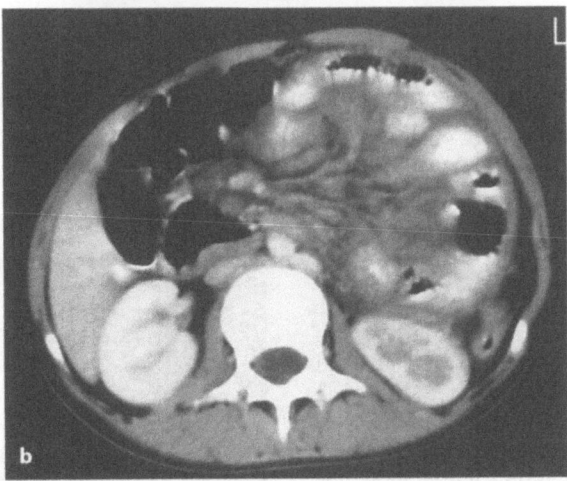

Fig. 3.2a,b. Peritoneal tuberculosis (fibrotic type). Transverse US image of the abdomen shows an adjoining matted loop of small bowels with loculated ascites (**a**). Corresponding CT image (**b**)

Ultrasound features are not pathognomonic of tuberculosis in the peritoneum, but, in the appropriate clinical setting, they may strongly suggest the diagnosis.

Ultrasound often shows free or loculated ascites (60–100% of cases); the ascites commonly contains fine, freely mobile septa composed of fibrin. However, it may occasionally be anechoic (Fig. 3.3).

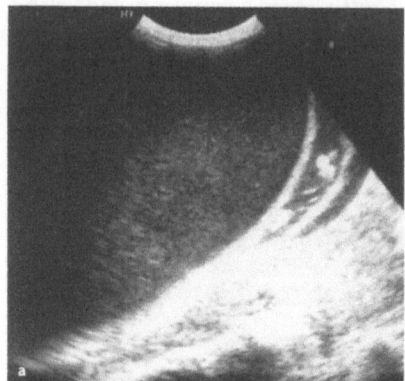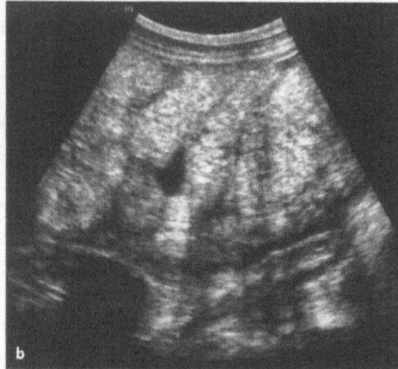

Fig. 3.3a,b. Peritoneal tuberculosis (wet type). Sonogram shows free ascites containing fine echoes (**a**) and loculated anechoic fluid between the bowels (**b**)

Irregular or nodular thickening of the peritoneum, omentum, and mesentery are other commonly encountered features of tuberculosis in the peritoneum (Fig. 3.4).

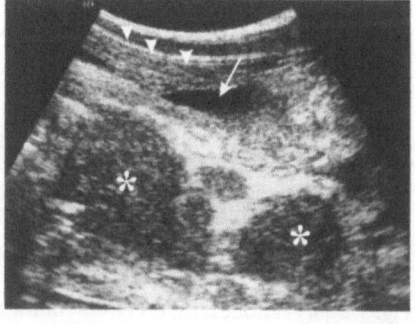

Fig. 3.4. Peritoneal and lymphadenitis tuberculosis. US transverse scan of abdomen shows thickening of the peritoneum (*arrowheads*), loculated ascites (*arrow*), and multiple lymph nodes (*asterisk*)

Fixed loops of bowel and mesentery standing out as spokes which radiate out the mesenteric root are described as the ultrasound "stellate" sign.

Ultrasound may be used as guidance for paracentesis and aspiration of enlarged lymph nodes for culture and cytologic study. It may be very helpful for the follow-up of the patients.

3.1.1.5
Lymph Node Tuberculosis

Lymphadenopathy is the most common manifestation of abdominal tuberculosis. Mesenteric, omental, periportal, and peripancreatic lymphatic groups are most commonly affected.

Lymphadenopathy may be discrete or conglomerated, due to periadenitis. Caseation may give rise to a hypoechoic center within the nodal mass. A similar appearance may occur in necrotizing metastatic nodes. However, diagnosis of tuberculous lymphadenitis should be considered in the appropriate clinical setting (Fig. 3.5).

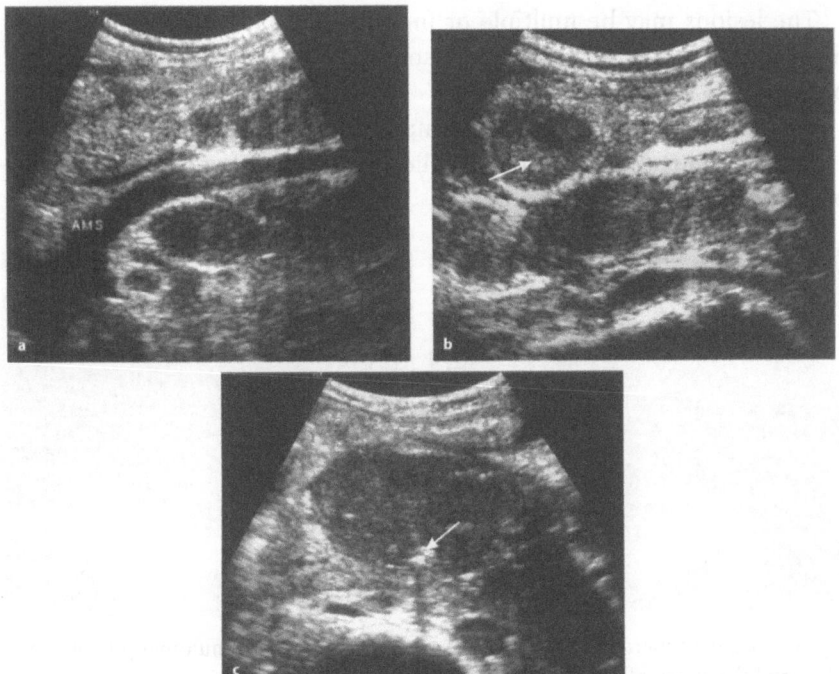

Fig. 3.5a–c. Abdominal tuberculous lymphadenitis. US images show mesenteric lymph node involvement. The necrotizing center of lymph nodes apparently anechoic (*arrow*, b) and their calcified feature (*arrow*, c) are suggestive of tuberculosis

Calcifications or heterogeneous echotexture of infected nodes before treatment are also suggestive of tuberculosis.

Lymph node masses, even when large, rarely cause obstruction of biliary tract, ureters, or bowel.

3.1.1.6
Hepatosplenic Tuberculosis

Hepatosplenic tuberculosis may be micronodular or macronodular.

The micronodular lesions are observed in the miliary form of pulmonary tuberculosis and usually present as moderate homogeneous or heterogeneous hepatosplenomegaly.

The liver and the spleen may show normal echogenicity or a hypoechoic pattern, giving rise to the "bright appearance" (Fig. 3.6).

Macronodular form of hepatosplenic tuberculosis is also called pseudo-tumoral tuberculosis or tuberculoma.

The lesions may be multiple or unique. Multiple lesions are well delineated, often hypoechoic on ultrasound, and scattered throughout the organ (Fig. 3.7).

The lesions may be hyperechoic and sometimes calcified.

Percutaneous aspiration biopsy allows histopathological confirmation of the diagnosis.

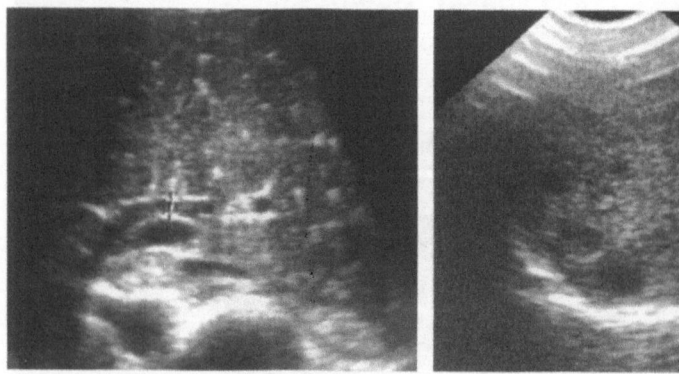 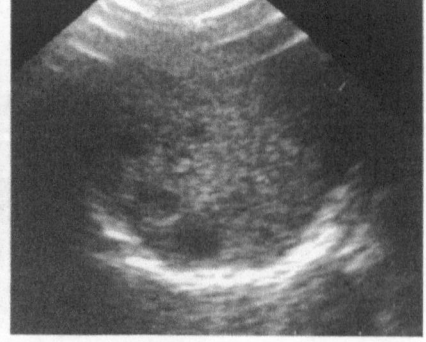

Fig. 3.6. Hepatic tuberculosis (miliary form). Multiple small granulomas giving rise to the "bright" pattern of the liver

Fig. 3.7. Tuberculosis of the spleen. US shows multiple hypoechoic nodules scattered in the spleen without splenomegaly

3.1.1.7
Tuberculosis of the Pancreas

Tuberculosis of the pancreas is extremely rare, especially when isolated.

Tuberculosis lesions in the pancreas are usually located in the head and, less commonly, in the body and tail.

Solitary lesions of pancreatic tuberculosis are seen as a hypoechoic well-defined mass, sometimes with calcification

Ultrasound rarely shows a diffuse enlargement of pancreas. Peripancreatic lymph nodes are sometimes detected.

3.1.1.8
Urogenital Tuberculosis

Urogenital tuberculosis is the second most frequent location of tuberculosis, after pulmonary involvement.

Ultrasound has less performance than intravenous pyelography and computed tomography (CT) scan in the diagnosis of renal tuberculosis.

Ultrasound is contributive in the advanced stage of the disease and particularly in the case of nonfunctional kidney.

Ultrasound may show:

- focal heterogenities of renal parenchyma
- pseudocystic lesions corresponding to caverns in the parenchyma or dilated calices (pyocalyx, see Fig. 2.64).

Hydronephrosis, in association with the typical aspect of coarctate pelvis, strongly suggests tuberculosis.

- parenchymal calcifications associated with granulomatous masses or in the late stage of the disease (Fig. 3.8).

In *tuberculous cystitis*, ultrasound may show a nonspecific thickening of the bladder wall, with reduced capacity.

At transrectal ultrasound, the most common finding of *tuberculous prostatitis* is the presence of hypoechoic areas, with an irregular pattern in the peripheral zone of the prostate.

Tuberculous orchitis usually manifests at ultrasonography as focal or diffuse areas of decreased echogenicity.

Tuberculous epididymitis evolves in a chronic way and appears as hyperechoic enlarged epididymis with macrocalcifications.

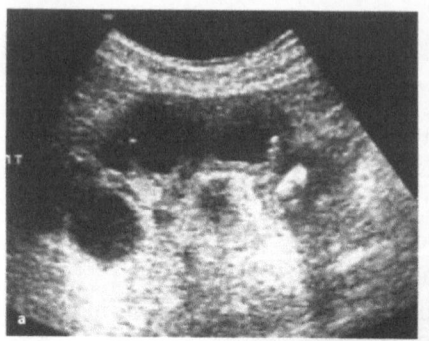
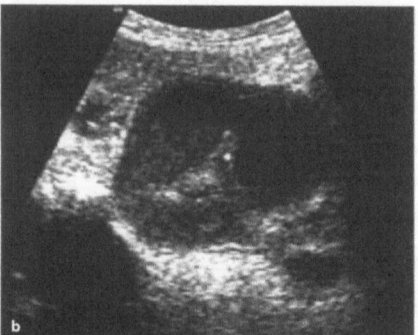
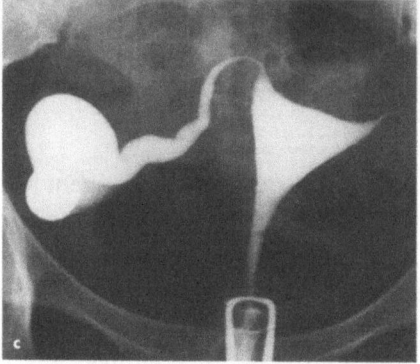

Fig. 3.8a–c. Urogenital tuberculosis. US demonstrates parenchymal abnormalities of the right kidney with pseudocystic lesions and focal calcification (**a**). The involvement of the right Fallopian tube gives rise to hydrosalpinx visualized by US (**b**) and by hysterosalpingography (**c**)

Tuberculosis of female genital tract can affect the Fallopian tubes, endometrium, and ovaries. Ultrasound may reveal pelvic extension of the disease and tubo-ovarian abscesses.

3.1.1.9
Peripheral Lymph Node Tuberculosis

Lymphatic tuberculosis is more common among children. Cervical or supraclavicular nodes are most commonly involved.

The ultrasound pattern is similar to that of abdominal lymphadenitis (see above).

3.1.1.10
Breast Tuberculosis

Tuberculosis involvement of the breast is rare and mostly secondary to extramammary tuberculous lesions.

The disease spreads to the breast by the lymphatic system, the blood, or due to contiguity from the pleura or thoracic wall.

Ultrasound findings are nonspecific, appearing as nodular mass, solid or cystic, mimicking benign or malignant tumors.

Both the findings of well circumscribed hypoechoic mass with moving internal echoes and the possible view of fistulae to the chest wall or pleura are highly suggestive of the diagnosis (Fig. 3.9).

Ultrasound-guided fine-needle aspiration biopsy can be easily performed for cytological and microbiological research.

Percutaneous drainage of breast tuberculous abscess is a noninvasive alternative to surgery and should be associated with antituberculous chemotherapy.

Ultrasound is also used in the follow-up of patients.

3.1.1.11
Tuberculous Soft Tissue Involvement

Tuberculous abscess formation may develop anywhere in the body. Nevertheless, such formations are frequently visualized near tuberculous osteitis or osteoarthritis, for example in the paravertebral region or iliopsoas muscle if the patient suffers from Potts' disease (tuberculous spondylitis), or in thoracic wall, if ribs are involved, etc. (Fig. 3.10).

Calcification within the abscess is highly suggestive of tuberculosis.

Ultrasound- and CT-guided percutaneous drainage contribute to the treatment, in conjunction with antituberculous drugs.

3.2
Viral Infections

3.2.1
AIDS and Sonography
(by Marcello Caremani, Danilo Tacconi, Alessandra Caremani)

In the HAART era, in both industrialized and underdeveloped countries, we deal with patients with HIV infection in:

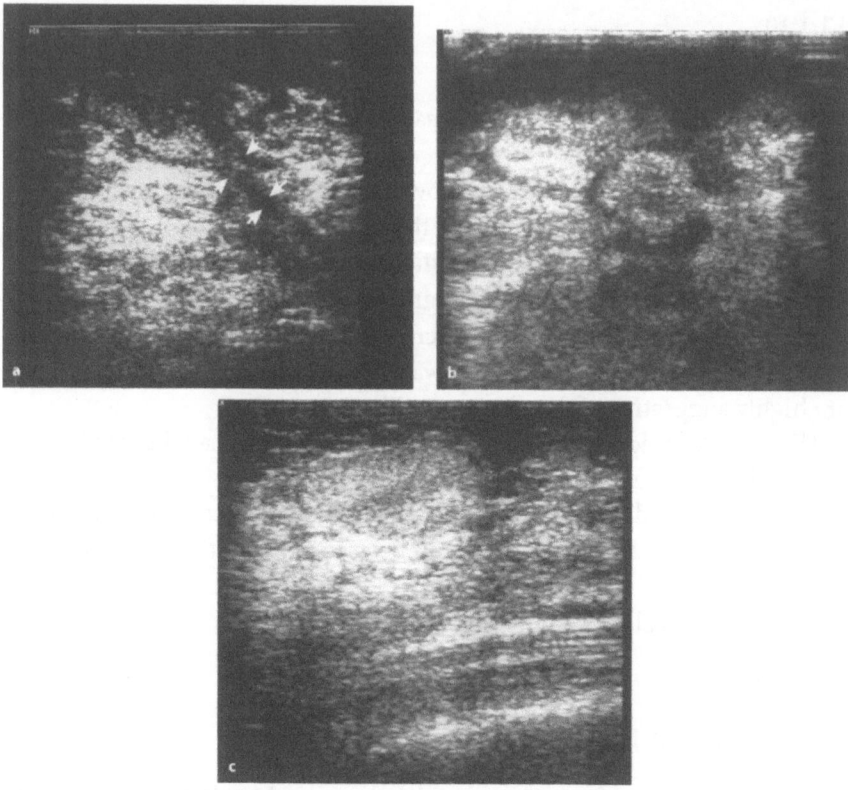

Fig. 3.9a–c. Tuberculosis of breast. (a) Sonogram shows a large hypoechoic heterogeneous area and a fistula connecting the lesion with retromammary region (*arrowheads*). (b) In another patient, the lesion is shown as anechoic pseudocystic area in the phase of abscess. (c) Another US pattern of tuberculous breast involvement is the pseudonodular form. Sonogram shows in this case a well delineated hyperechoic mass

Fig. 3.10. Psoas abscess seen in tuberculous spondylodiscitis. Sonogram shows a large hypoechoic collection in right psoas muscle

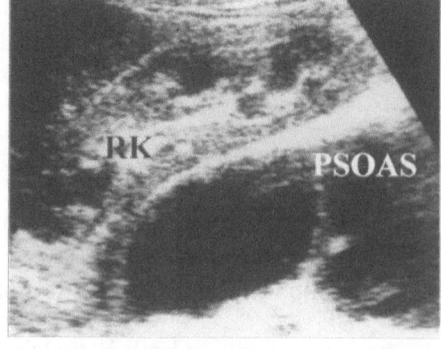

1. Virological remission and immune recovery
2. New infections with delayed diagnosis and severe immune deficiency
3. Progression of the disease because of viral resistance and thus immune deficiency

Therefore, many patients with HIV infection/AIDS still require a diagnostic imaging examination because of the presence of infections or opportunistic neoplastic pathologies.

Ultrasound (US) is a first-level imaging method because of its sensitivity and specificity, particularly in abdominal pathology. In fact, abdominal pathology is second only to pulmonary pathology, and it seems more frequent in the HAART era, since antiretroviral treatment and therapy of opportunistic infections (OIs) have increased the survival of patients with HIV infection.

However, the abdominal manifestations of acquired immune deficiency syndrome are proteiform and tend to involve several anatomical regions. In most cases, the lesions are aspecific organomegalies and rarely echostructural alterations of parenchyma or systems. Therefore, the ultrasound examination does not often give a suggestive picture, also because OI and AIDS-related neoplasias can produce similar ultrasound aspects.

However, there are anatomical-ultrasound correlations in AIDS patients. Granulomatous lesions, generally caused by CMV, mycobacteria, and Mycetes, increase the parenchymal echogenicity, whereas necrotic lesions, caused by bacteria, mycobacteria, and fungi produce roundish hypoechogenic alterations.

Lymphomas often present a nodular hypoechogenic aspect, whereas Kaposi's sarcoma (KS), which usually spreads via a perivascular path, causes an increase of echogenicity and, thus, iso-hyperechogenic lesions.

In the pre-HAART era, the patient with HIV infection/AIDS arrived at ultrasound because of increased transaminase and/or hepatomegaly (22–27%), abdominal pain (20%), fever (11%) and diarrhea (3%).

In the HAART era, abdominal pain and fever are the most frequent symptoms that cause the patient to undergo an ultrasound examination, followed by diarrhea and hepatic pathology from co-infection by HIV/HCV.

Pain still presents an incidence of 15%, whereas HIV- related disease is responsible for 65%, but the diagnosis is made at autopsy in 33% of cases.

The most frequent causes are HIV-related cholangitis, pancreatitis, and complications of neoplasias during AIDS.

The incidence of HIV-related cholangitis varies according to the case study, ranging from 1% to 20%; it can cause a pathology involving only the intra- and extrahepatic biliary pathways and/or cholecystitis.

The etiopathogenesis is still uncertain, since both immune deficiency and HIV and opportunistic infections are taken into consideration (*Cryptosporidium*/microsporids 30–40%, CMV 20%, MAC 5–6%, *Candida*, *Salmonella*)

In addition to pain (present in 60–65% of cases), there is fever (77.14%), nausea and vomiting (57.7%), and a positive Murphy's sign (54.7%).

The sonographic signs of acute alithiasic cholecystitis are:

1. Thickening of the cholecystic wall: > 3 mm, with a three-layered appearance (two echogenic interfaces separated by a hypoechogenic line)
2. Distension of the gall bladder with sludge in its interior
3. Sonographic Murphy's sign
4. Collection of pericholecystic liquid (Fig. 3.11)

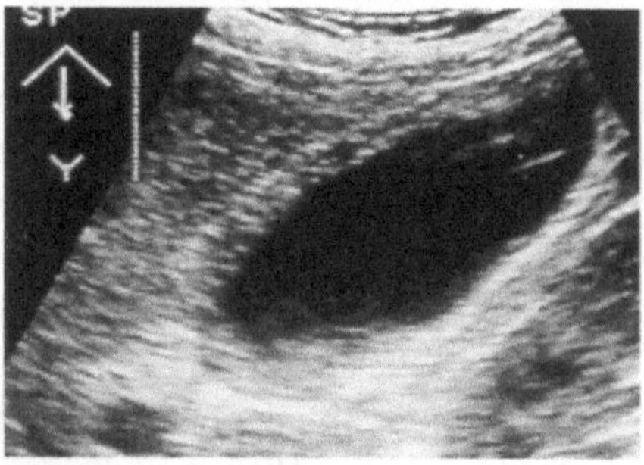

Fig. 3.11. Acute HIV-related cholecystitis. Large cholecyst with three-layered appearance of the wall and the presence of stratified sludge posteriorly

The sonographic signs of cholangitis are:

1. Sectorial dilatation of the intrahepatic VB, associated with hyperechogenic thickening of the periportal area (fibrosis)
2. Hypoechogenic halo surrounding the VB (edema)
3. Dilatation of the VBP (odditis)
4. Hyperechogenic thickening of the VBP (Fig. 3.12)

The sensitivity (97%) and specificity (100%) of ultrasound are high, with a diagnostic accuracy that reaches 98%. Nevertheless, it is often necessary to make a differential diagnosis with edema of the gall bladder during dysproteinemia and acute hepatitis, whereas for cholangitis with lithiasis

Fig. 3.12. Right oblique subcostal scan, showing a clear sectorial dilatation of a biliary branch (*arrows*) due to HIV-related cholangitis

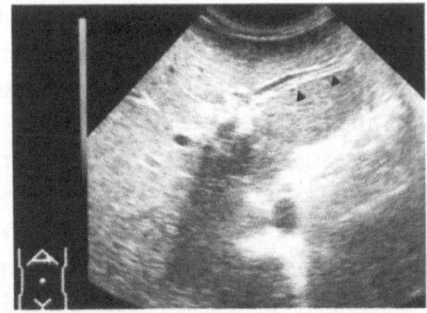

and other causes of biliary pathway obstruction, pancreatitis and sclerosing cholangitis secondary to other causes should be considered.

Pancreatitis in a patient with HIV infection/AIDS can be secondary to opportunistic infections (CMV, MAC, cryptosporids) and drugs, but is more severe than the forms affecting HIV-negative patients.

Ultrasound has low sensitivity in this pathology, especially in the initial forms (17.5%), but improves when the pancreatic necrosis exceeds 33%. In the initial phase, there may be an increase in volume and in echostructure, and sometimes sectorial or diffuse hypoechogenicity.

In the advanced phase, the hypoechogenicity is very evident and is associated with irregular and blurred contours and the presence of peri-pancreatic collections, even up to a true ascites (Fig. 3.13).

Fever is the most frequent cause of admission, with difficulty of diagnosis in 10–20% of patients with HIV/AIDS; OIs are responsible in 80–90% of cases and lymphomas in 4–10%; the cause remains unknown in 5–8% of cases.

Fig. 3.13. Right and transverse subcostal scans. Pancreas with increased volume and diffuse hypoechogenicity (*arrows*) due to pancreatitis caused by HIV-related CMV infection

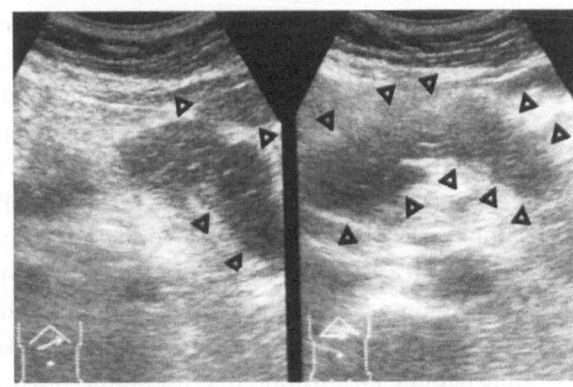

Hepatic and/or splenic abscesses, tubercular, mycotic or *Pneumocystis* localization in these organs, lymphomas, cholangitis, and enterocolitis are the main causes of the fever, often associated with pain starting from the abdomen.

Abscesses of the liver and spleen are most frequently caused by Mycetes (*Pneumocystis*, *Cryptococcus*, *Aspergillus*, and *Candida*), less often by mycobacteria (*Mycobacterium hominis* and MAC), bacteria (*Bartonella*, *Rhodococcus*, *Nocardia*, *Staphylococcus*), and protozoans.

In hepatosplenic abscesses caused by fungi, ultrasound shows lesions with a characteristic aspect, such as the wheel inside a wheel, or less specific ones, such as target lesions and roundish hypoechogenic lesions. (Fig. 3.14).

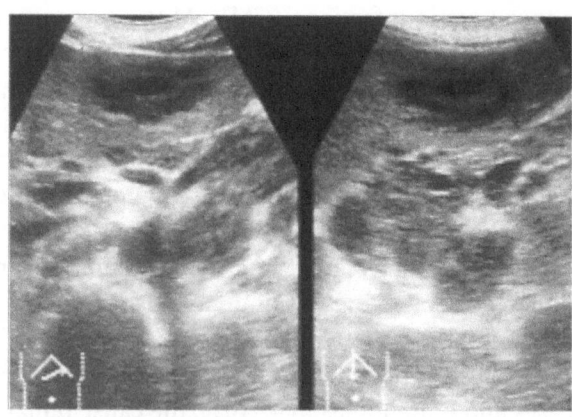

Fig. 3.14. Right and longitudinal oblique subcostal scan. Wheel inside a wheel lesion of the left lobe of the liver due to an hepatic abscess and abdominal lymphoadenomegaly caused by *Cryptococcus* in an AIDS patient

Abdominal pneumocystosis can cause a specific organomegaly, sometimes associated with multiple hyperechogenic spots (Fig. 3.15) or diffuse hyperechogenicity (snowstorm-like), sometimes associated with ascites.

Tubercular localization in the liver and spleen can cause a homogeneous organomegaly, as well as diffuse hyperechogenicity with snowstorm-like aspect, small roundish hypoechogenic lesions with and without a wall, calcifications, ascites, and peritoneal thickening (Fig. 3.16).

Lymphomas in patients with HIV infection/AIDS present peculiar characteristics, since, in most cases, they have the B-phenotype, with a high degree of malignancy, frequently extranodal and in atypical sites, with onset in an advanced phase and with high aggressiveness.

While hepatic localization of lymphomas during AIDS does not exceed 8%, splenic localization can reach 15%; in both these organs, as well as in

Fig. 3.15. Right oblique subcostal scan. Diffuse hyperechogenicity of the liver with snowstorm-like aspect due to hepatic localization of *Pneumocystis carinii*

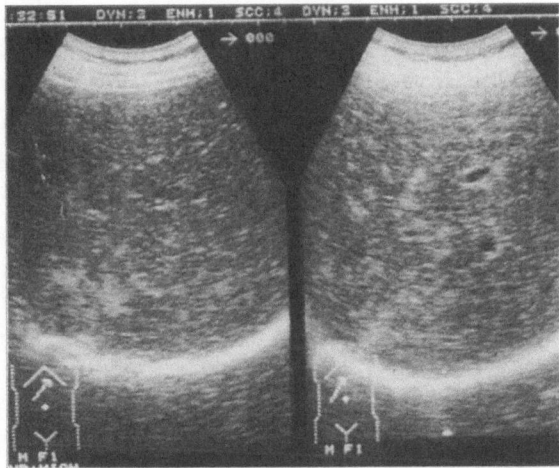

Fig. 3.16. Left intercostal scan in a patient in right lateral decubitus. Spleen with increased volume and inhomogeneous due to the presence of numerous hypoechogenic formations caused by tubercular localization during AIDS

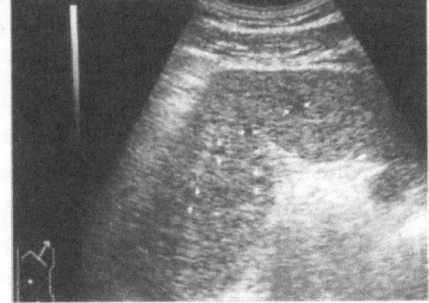

the pancreas and kidney, they present as hypoechoic nodular lesions with irregular and blurred contours, sometimes with diffuse hypoechogenicity (Fig. 3.17).

In the pre-HAART era, lymphomatous localization in the gastrointestinal apparatus was the cause of death in 8–10% of cases, with an autopsy incidence of 15% and an incidence of 4–28%, second only to localizations in the bone marrow and central nervous system (CNS).

In these patients, ultrasound often shows particular appearances, characterized by hypo-hyperechogenic thickenings with a bridging layer sign type (as an bridging aspect), sometimes with pseudorenal aspects (frequently at the gastric level), a wheel aspect, or hypoechogenic lesions and complex mass images.

A peculiar aspect is present in patients with lymphoma of the serous cavity (body cavity B-lymphoma); it presents with ascites and hypo-

Fig. 3.17. Right oblique subcostal scan. Liver altered by the presence of two roundish hypoechogenic lesions (*arrows*) due to hepatic localization of an NH lymphoma in a patient with HIV infection/AIDS

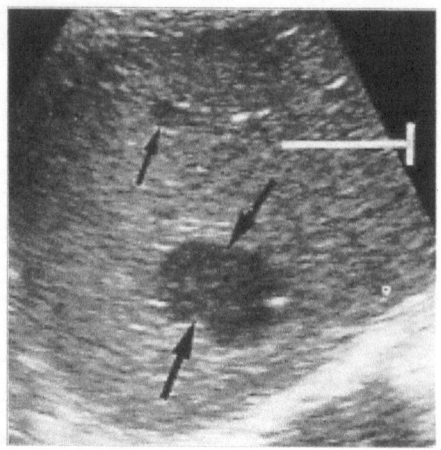

hyperechogenic thickening of the serosa of the small intestine and colon, making the layers composing the intestinal loops very visible (Fig. 3.18).

Abdominal lymph node pathology is very frequent in patients with HIV infection, affecting more than 50% of them; however, the size is less than 25 mm in 90% of cases, generally due to HIV- and/or HCV-related reactive hyperplasia.

The abdominal lymph nodes are only visible if increased in volume. In lymphomatous pathology, they present as roundish hypo-anechogenic lesions with disappearance or shifting of the hilus sign, associated with echostructural inhomogeneity and alteration of the contours. The presence of hypoechogenic or inhomogeneous polylobate masses is not infrequent.

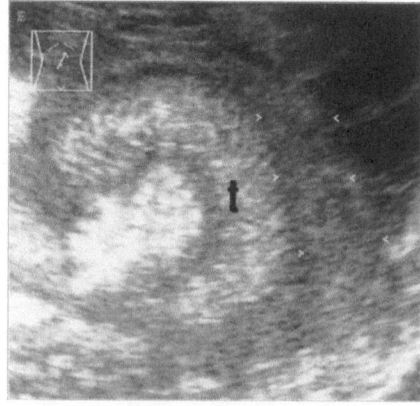

Fig. 3.18. Oblique paraumbilical scan. The small intestine (t) presents thickening (*arrows*) of the peritoneal wall with a inhomogeneous aspect and irregular and blurred contours. Lymphoma of the serous cavity in a patient with AIDS

The differential diagnosis with forms secondary to OI can be difficult, since both pathologies can present the same size, a longitudinal diameter/inferior diameter ratio less than 2 (long axis/short axis ratio < 2), disappearance or shifting of the hilus sign, echostructural inhomogeneity, and irregularity of the contours.

In the pre-HAART era, the incidence of diarrhea in patients with HIV infection/AIDS ranged from 20% to 40%, and today it still varies according to the case study and degree of immune deficiency; this symptom is caused by OI, neoplasias, HIV-related enteropathy, and drugs (this is currently the most frequent cause of diarrhea in patients on antiretroviral therapy).

In most cases, ultrasound is unable to reveal specific signs of pathology, but may indicate the presence of a non-neoplastic gastrointestinal involvement.

In infectious diarrhea, ultrasound shows five sonographic patterns in 80% of cases:

1. Dilated intestinal loops occupied by liquid, associated with hyper-peristalsis: a frequent sonographic pattern in diarrhea secondary to HIV-related enteropathy and in diarrhea caused by drugs.
2. Sectorial or diffuse thickening of the walls of the small intestine and/or colon: a sonographic pattern present in both the HIV-related form and during opportunistic infections.
3. Crohn-like lesions, characterized by thickening and disappearance of the sonographic signs of the intestinal walls of the small intestine and colon: a typical finding in OI.

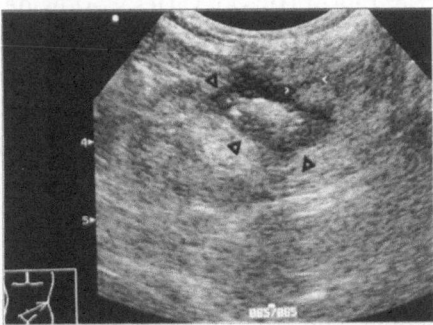

Fig. 3.19. Oblique scan passing through the left inferior quadrant of the abdomen. Presence of a pseudorenal image with irregular and blurred contours (*black arrows*), giving rise to a hypoechogenic line that passes deeply into the peritoneal fat (*white arrows*). Colitis from CMV penetrating into the peritoneal fat in an AIDS patient

4. Pseudotumoral lesions, sometimes with pseudorenal images: a frequent finding in CMV infections of the colon.
5. Associated findings: ascites and signs of perforation (Fig. 3.19).

3.2.1.1
Conclusions

The AIDS emergency has ended in industrialized countries, but is still a serious health problem in many underdeveloped countries.

Pathologies related to HIV and immune deficiency often require a flexible diagnostic imaging technique with high diagnostic accuracy, such as sonography, which can shorten and simplify the diagnostic-therapeutic pathway.

3.2.2
Viral Hepatitis
(by Harald T. Lutz, Josef Deuerling)

3.2.2.1
Epidemiology

Hepatitis A occurs sporadically or epidemically around the world. An especially high prevalence is seen in Africa, the Middle East, parts of southeast Russia, and middle America.

Hepatitis B is spread largely by whole blood and its products, semen and saliva. The carrier rate of HBs-Ag varies worldwide between less than 2% in North America, western Europe, Australia, and New Zealand, 2–7% in southern Europe, central Asia and Russia, Japan, and parts of South America, and more than 8% in the high-risk areas such as Southeast Asia, the Middle East, Africa, and the Amazon region in South America.

Acute Hepatitis D is also a worldwide disease, but has an especially high prevalence in some Mediterranean countries, Arabic countries, and East Africa as well as in the region of the Amazon.

The prevalence of Hepatitis C is again lower in northern countries and high in southern regions, and especially in some areas of the Pacific.

Hepatitis E is more common in areas with low sanitary standards.

Other viral infections affecting the liver are the *Epstein-Barr virus*, mainly in young adults, the *Cytomegalovirus*, and the *Herpes simplex virus*, mainly in immunosuppressed patients, Lassa fever (*Arenavirus*) in West

Africa, the *Ebola virus* in some African countries, and yellow fever in central parts of Africa.

3.2.2.2
Pathology

The pathologies of the various virus infections of the liver are more or less identical: hepatic cell necrosis is associated with cellular infiltration. In severe cases, necrosis may be confluent and whole lobules may be involved. In cases of fulminant hepatitis, the liver size is reduced and the capsule becomes irregular. If the patient survives, a nodular regeneration is seen after 2–3 weeks.

In the chronic stage of hepatitis, mononuclear cells accumulate in nodular form within the lobule parenchyma and the portal triads. In active chronic hepatitis, piecemeal necrosis is present and may lead to bridging necrosis. Connective tissue membranes are seen as perilobular fibrosis and may stretch from one portal triad to the next. Over the years, the connective tissue will develop to a hepatic fibrosis in the beginning, without disturbance of the lobule architecture.

With the alteration of the lobule structure in the progress of chronic hepatitis and the presence of regenerative nodules, the stage of posthepatitic cirrhosis has developed. Following these typical alterations, portal hypertension occurs.

The risk of eventually developing hepatocellular carcinoma (HCC) is very high in patients with hepatitis B and C virus infection. With a high incidence in southeast Asia and parts of Africa, HCC is one of the most common malignant tumors worldwide.

3.2.2.3
Ultrasound Findings

In the acute stage of viral hepatitis and even in the beginning of a fulminant hepatitis, ultrasound shows an almost normal liver, which may sometimes be slightly but not significant enlarged. The echo pattern is normal, too. The "centrilobular pattern" described by several authors as a more echo-poor pattern of the parenchyma and striking bright echoes from the wall of the portal vein branches can be seen in healthy subjects as well (Fig. 3.20).

The lymph nodes in the hepato-duodenal ligament may be enlarged with a more echo-rich pattern (Fig. 3.21). The gall bladder may be slightly

Fig. 3.20. Acute viral hepatitis. The liver is not enlarged. The so-called "centrilobular pattern" with an echo-poor parenchyma and bright echoes from the vessels is demonstrated in this case

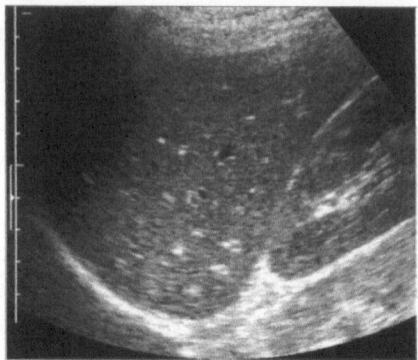

Fig. 3.21. Acute viral hepatitis C. Slightly enlarged lymph nodes are seen, in the ligament in front of the caval vein

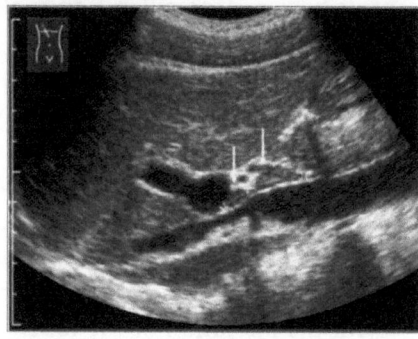

enlarged, with a normal or sometimes thickened wall, as a sign of malfunction.

In the latter stage of fulminant hepatitis, the size of the liver decreases and the surface became irregular.

In the regenerative stage of the fulminant hepatitis, the echo pattern becomes inhomogeneous due to shrunken and atrophic parts and nodular regenerative areas on the other side. These findings may vary highly, depending on the extent of necrosis and regeneration.

The liver of patients with chronic hepatitis usually looks quite normal, too (Figs. 3.22, 3.23). Only in the late stage, the liver may be slightly enlarged and the lower edge may be rounded. The surface still remains smooth (Fig. 3.24). A more echo-rich pattern, caused by the fatty content, may sometimes be seen. In these cases, one must consider additional disorders of the liver, e.g., by alcohol, existing simultaneously.

Enlarged lymph nodes in the hepato-duodenal ligament may be demonstrated especially in the chronic stage of HCV-associated hepatitis. Whether this indicates a more severe disease or has any importance concerning the prognosis and the treatment is still in discussion.

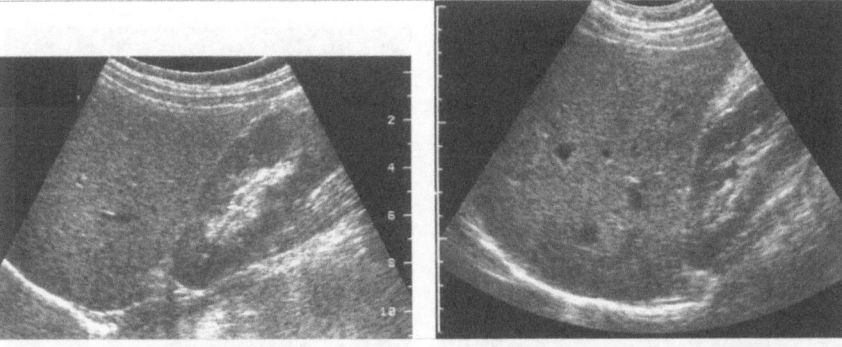

Fig. 3.22. Chronic viral hepatitis. The liver looks quite normal. Histology: highly active

Fig. 3.23. Chronic viral hepatitis. Inconspicuous finding. Histology: low activity

Fig. 3.24. Chronic viral hepatitis C. Only the rounded edge is conspicuous. Histology: high activity

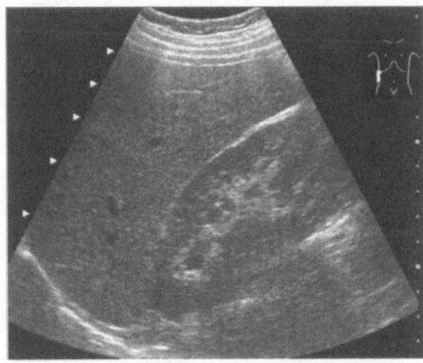

In the late stage of the virus hepatitis, the signs of cirrhosis become visible (Figs. 3.25–3.28):

- shrinkage of the whole liver and especially of the right lobe
- hypertrophy of the caudate lobe (ratio caudate lobe/right lobe > 0.65)
- irregular surface (the most sensitive sonographic symptom)
- inhomogeneous, coarse echo pattern
- signs of portal hypertension

The ultrasonic findings in portal hypertension are not very conspicuous and significant in the early stage. Dilatation of the portal vein is an especially unreliable and late symptom.

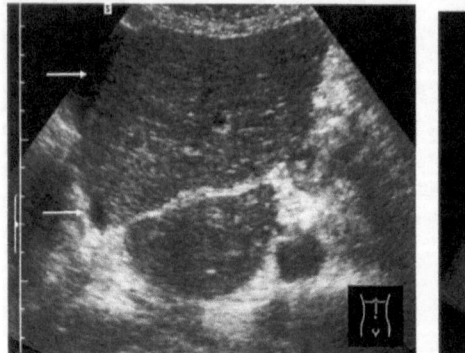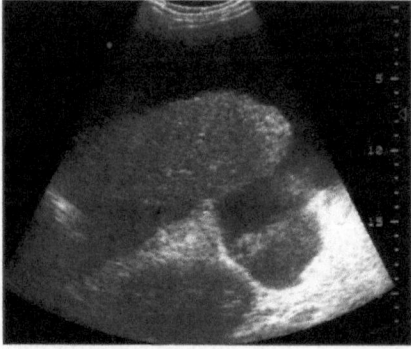

Fig. 3.25. Chronic viral hepatitis. Liver enlarged, rounded edge. Histology: highly aggressive, transition to cirrhosis

Fig. 3.26. Posthepatitic liver cirrhosis. The liver is slightly enlarged; the echo pattern is not conspicuous; the edge is rounded and the surface is not absolutely smooth. Only the ascites is really suspicious of cirrhosis

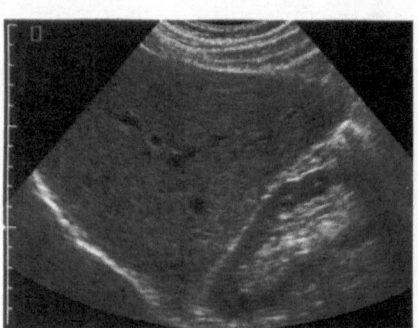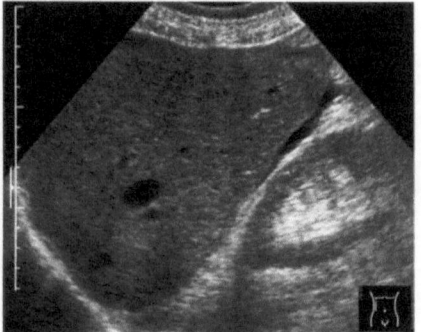

Fig. 3.27. Liver cirrhosis. Note the enlarged caudate lobe and the coarse echo pattern. *Arrows* mark a small line of ascites

Fig. 3.28. Liver cirrhosis. The liver is shrunken; the surface is irregular; high amount of ascites: late stage of posthepatitic cirrhosis

Sonographic signs of portal hypertension are (Figs. 3.29–3.33): B-scan:

– diameter of portal vein > 14 mm
– rigid caliber during Valsalva's maneuver
– round cross-section of the portal vein (normally oval)
– portal vein thrombosis
– collaterals

Fig. 3.29. Portal hypertension. Note the dilated portal vein and the recanalized umbilical vein (*arrows*)

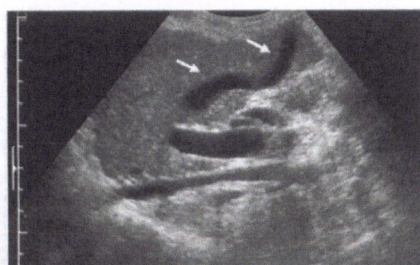

Fig. 3.30. Recanalized paraumbilical veins. Sonographic equivalent of the so-called "Caput Medusae"

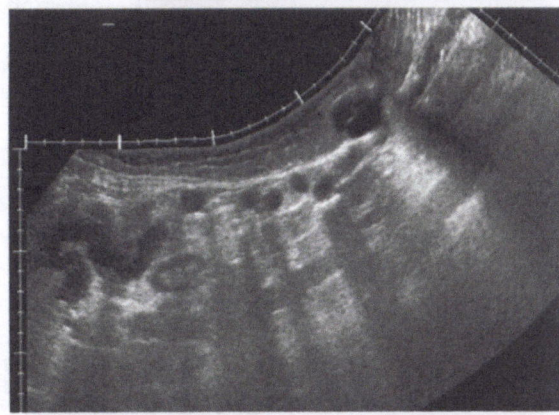

Fig. 3.31. Portal hypertension. Reduced flow in the dilated portal vein

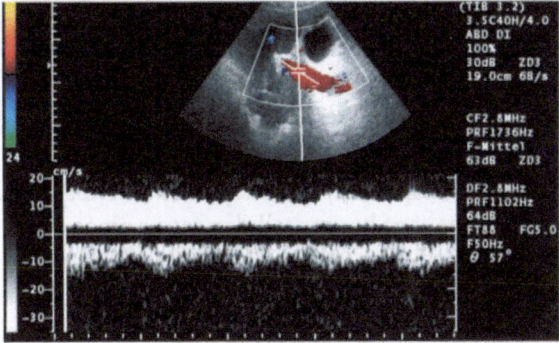

- ascites
- splenomegaly

Doppler Technique:

- reduced flow in the portal vein
- reversed flow in the portal vein
- flow signals in the paraumbilical vein inside the ligamentum teres
- high resistance index (RI > 0.61) in the branches of the splenic artery

Fig. 3.32. Portal hypertension. Reversed, hepatofugal flow in the portal vein

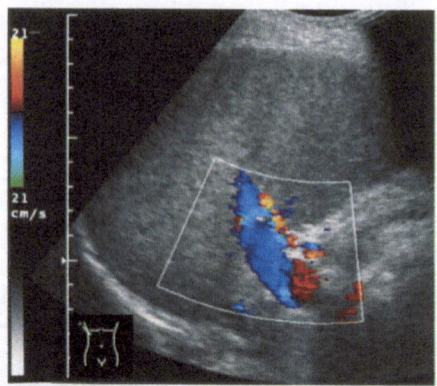

Fig. 3.33. Portal hypertension. High resistance index (RI) in the splenic artery (RI = 0.85)

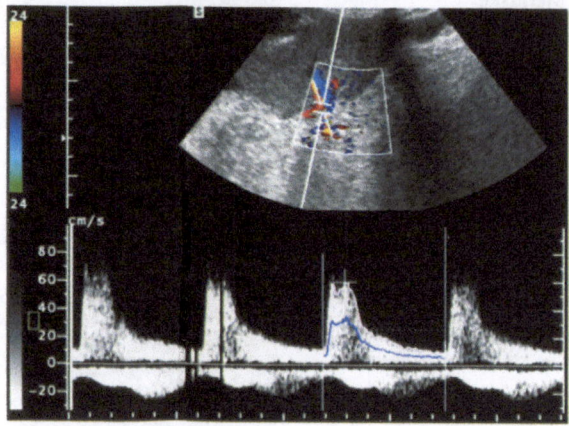

Cirrhosis, especially posthepatitic cirrhosis, means a high risk for the development of hepatocellular carcinomas (HCCs). Thus, in patients with known cirrhosis, ultrasonic examination must always include a careful search for focal lesions.

In most cases, HCC is seen as a solitary lesion. The echo pattern of these tumors varies widely, ranging from echo-poor (small) nodules or even echo-free (necrosis) lesions to tumors with echo-rich or target-like patterns and completely inhomogeneous lesions.

In many hepatocellular carcinomas, a typical hypervascularity can be demonstrated by using sensitive color Doppler techniques. Currently, the best way to demonstrate the typical hypervascularity is with the use of intravenous contrast agents. This technique enables the exact differentiation between HCC and regenerative nodules, which may sometimes be difficult with the gray-scale technique (Figs. 3.34, 3.35a–c). Metastatic liver tumors, on the other hand, are very rare in cirrhotic liver.

Fig. 3.34. Liver cirrhosis, regenerative nodule (32 mm). Not the low contrast of the nodule and the irregular surface of the left hepatic lobe

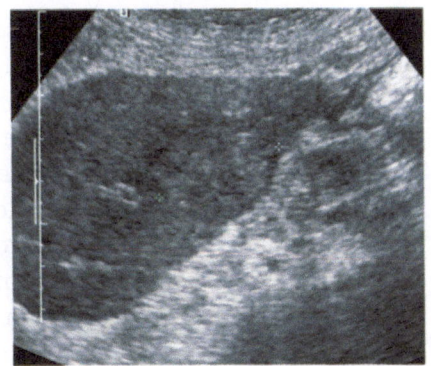

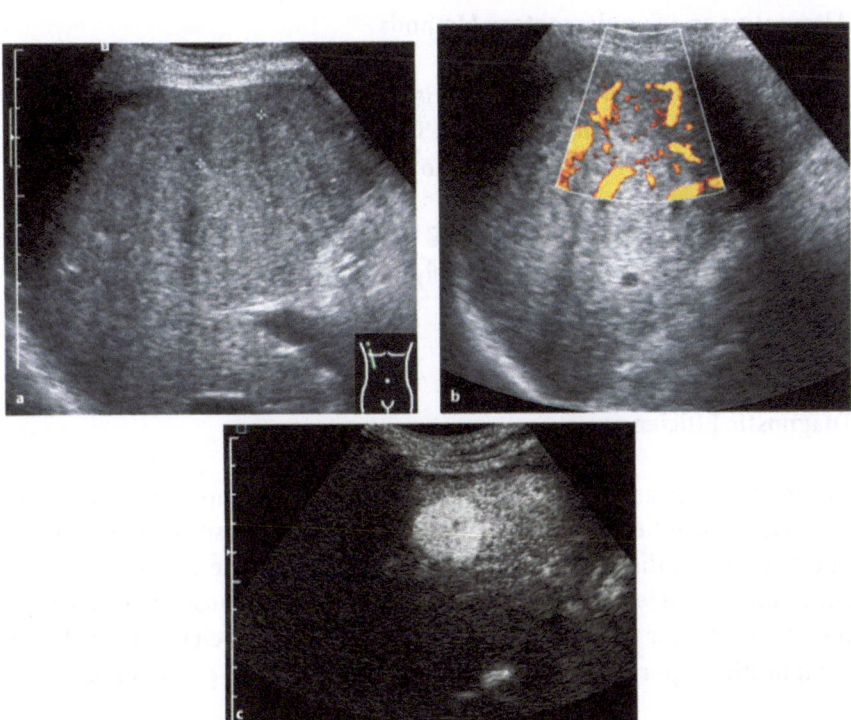

Fig. 3.35a–c. Hepatocellular carcinoma. B-scan: the focal lesion (27 mm) in the cirrhotic liver shows low contrast and a halo, similar to the regenerative nodule, seen in Fig. 3.34 (**a**). Power Doppler: no proof of hypervascularity (**b**). Contrast: typical highly positive contrast in the early stage after 20 sec (**c**)

3.2.2.4
Differential Diagnosis

The ultrasonic findings described are at no stage typical of a virus hepatitis. In the acute and early chronic stages, the liver looks quite normal. The reliable ultrasonic diagnosis of cirrhosis, on the other hand, does not give any indication of the etiology of the disease.

Enlarged lymph nodes are seen more often in younger patients and, possibly, in Hepatitis C, but are again no marker for the type of the disease, nor the severity.

3.2.2.5
Alternative and Supplementary Methods

The diagnosis of acute virus hepatitis is usually established based on the clinical features and laboratory tests. The development of a chronic hepatitis can be suspected in light of laboratory test results, but must be confirmed finally by a biopsy.

The differentiation between HCC and regenerative nodules is possible with contrast media. Alternatively, an ultrasonically guided biopsy is suitable for this purpose.

3.2.2.6
Diagnostic Efficiency

In summary, ultrasound is of limited value in the diagnosis and the management of virus hepatitis. In the acute stage, it may be used to demonstrate or exclude other disorders, e.g., of the biliary tract. In the chronic stage, ultrasound is sufficient to detect the development of cirrhosis in most cases. It is also useful for the follow-up controls in the stage of cirrhosis, to detect complications, portal hypertension, and hepatocellular carcinoma.

3.2.3
Dengue Fever
(by Leandro J. Fernandez)

3.2.3.1
Overview

Dengue, the proper name is Dysgeusia, is an acute infectious disease caused by the Arbovirus (*Flaviviridae* family), which is common in the tropical and subtropical areas throughout the world, having its maximum incidence at the end of the rainy season. A significant increase in the incidence of this infectious disease has taken place in the last 20 years and, in 1998, it was deemed to be the most important tropical mosquito-transmitted infectious disease, surpassed only by malaria.

The disease includes two forms, classic dengue and hemorrhagic dengue or dengue shock syndrome, known as DHF-SSD.

Four serotypes have been identified for this virus (DEN1, DEN2, DEN3, DEN4), there being a scarce cross-immunity between the antibodies generated by these serotypes. As a result, when a person suffers from this disease, he/she becomes immune only to a specific serotype.

3.2.3.2
Epidemiology

Dengue is an endemic and epidemic disease in almost all of the tropical regions and in most subtropical regions. With an important incidence in Africa, it is more predominant in Southeast Asia, the Pacific Islands, and Central and South America. It has become a major health problem as endemic areas are inhabited by more than 2500 million people. It has been estimated that its annual incidence is 10 million cases per year for classic dengue and 500,000 cases for the hemorrhagic variety. Its mortality ranges from 1–5% for treated patients to a maximum of 50% for nontreated or poorly treated patients. In recent years, epidemic outbreaks have been reported in Thailand, China, India, Sri Lanka, Cuba, Puerto Rico, Brazil, and Venezuela. Furthermore, suspected imported cases have been reported in Spain, Germany, Italy, Israel, and the U.S.A. (Fig. 3.36).

The disease is transmitted by the mosquito species *Aedes aegypti*, which is the main vector, and the *Aedes albopictus* species (Fig. 3.37).

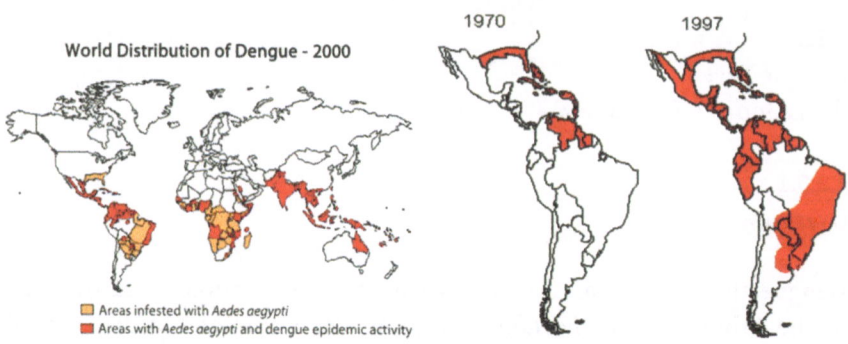

Fig. 3.36. Dengue fever distribution around the world

Fig. 3.37. Distribution of the transmitting mosquito Aedes in America, 1970 and 1997

3.2.3.3
Symptoms

Classic Dengue

The infection has an incubation period ranging from 3 to 14 days, its average period being 5–8 days. After this phase, a fever condition develops abruptly with temperatures in the 39–40 °C range, chill, heavy and widespread osteomuscular pain, especially in the lumbar region, neck and shoulders, as well as in the knees and hips. The disease is nicknamed 'breakbone fever' for these last two symptoms. Severe cephalgia and retro-ocular pain are also typical of this condition. Other associated symptoms are nausea, vomiting, epigastralgia, anorexia, weakness, deep depression, cutaneous hyperesthesia, and dysgeusia.

Initially, the fever lasts 2–3 days and, after that point, it stabilizes for two days. Then it begins a new 3–7-day cycle, but this time with a lower intensity. Between the third and fifth day, itching exanthema emerges that is very similar to measles, especially in the thorax, face, and limbs. This exanthema can cause desquamation. In addition to this, widespread adenopathy is frequently detected.

Hemorrhagic Dengue

The symptoms are similar to those of the classic form, but are also associated with bleeding with an intensity that varies depending on the severity of the clinical manifestations. These can include a positive tourniquet test with or without spontaneous bleeding, petechiae, purpura, epistaxis, and gingival and digestive hemorrhage.

Patients with DHF-SSD present hepatomegaly, polyadenopathy, and possibly splenomegaly, hypotension, hemodynamic instability, shock, disseminated intravascular coagulation, and massive gastrointestinal hemorrhage. Some unusual cases present with myocarditis, important pleural effusion, and encephalopathy.

The vast majority of patients overcoming either the classic or the hemorrhagic form of the disease remain in a considerably weak state for a period of several weeks.

3.2.3.4
Laboratory Findings

Findings include important leukopenia, with left deviation of the white cells formula, thrombocytopenia, mild elevation of transaminase levels and, in the most severe cases, effects on the coagulation tests, prolongation of PT and PTT. We have observed that thrombocytopenia is increased when fever disappears. Therefore, repeated platelet counts are required during this critical period. Elevation of hematocrit levels reveals hemoconcentration, which is an indication of the severity of manifestations. Serology is generally positive as of the fifth day after onset of disease.

3.2.3.5
Degrees of Clinical Severity

The severity of this disease falls into four degrees:

Degree I: Fever, general symptoms and positive tourniquet test
Degree II: Degree I plus spontaneous hemorrhage on the skin, gums, gastrointestinal tract, and other areas.
Degree III: Degree II plus circulatory shortage and agitation.
Degree IV: Shock. Nondetectable artery pressure.

In all phases, there is thrombocytopenia and hemoconcentration. Degrees III and IV are related to DHF-SSD.

3.2.3.6
Ultrasound Findings

Ultrasound techniques have been used for the evaluation of adults and children suffering from dengue. The reported findings in the literature considerably match our observations during the epidemic outbreaks in Venezuela from the mid-1990s to year 2001.

The reported changes vary according to the severity of each case. In adults with DHF Degree III, pleural effusion has been observed in 53% of cases, thickening of gall bladder walls in 43% (Fig. 3.38), and mild ascites in 15% of cases (Figs. 3.39, 3.40). Abdominal ultrasound was more sensitive than thoracic X-rays for the detection of pleural effusion.

In pediatric patients with Degree I-II disease, ultrasound findings are pleural effusion in 30% of cases, ascites in 34%, thickening of gall bladder walls in 32%, and pancreatic enlargement in 14% of cases. In Degree III and IV cases, reported findings are pleural effusion, ascites, and thickening of vesicular walls in 95% of cases, peri- and pararenal collections in 77% of cases, hepatomegaly 56%, pancreatic enlargement 44%, splenomegaly

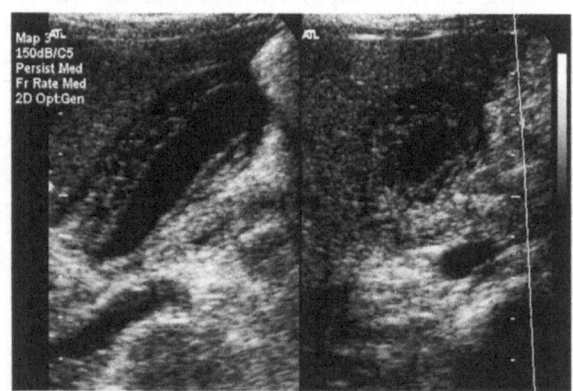

Fig. 3.38. Dengue fever: thickened gall bladder wall

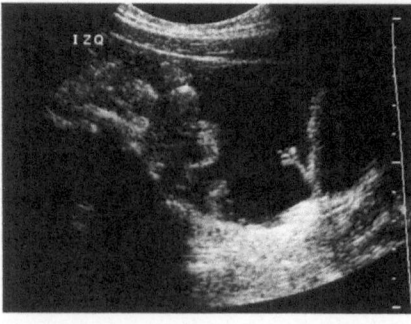
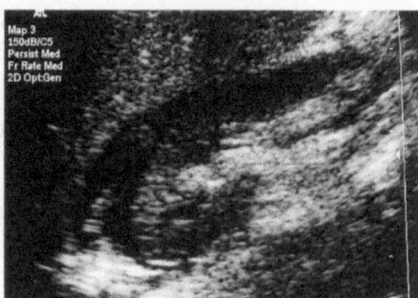

Fig. 3.39. Ascites in Dengue disease

Fig. 3.40. Small amount of ascites in a case of Dengue fever, demonstrated in Morrison's pouch

16%, hepatic or splenic subcapsular collections 9%, and pericardial effusion in 8% of cases.

An index was recently prepared based on ultrasound findings that has a shock-predictive value (DHF-SSD). The score is 0–12 as given by the ultrasound alterations observed (pleural effusion, liquid within the Morrison's pouch, thickening of gall bladder walls, etc.), with a "cut-off" a value of 5. Patients over this value have a higher risk of developing the most severe form of this disease. Based on these results, we can state that ultrasound can be useful in the estimation of severity of dengue fever.

3.3
Parasitic Diseases

3.3.1
Amebiasis
(by Leandro J. Fernandez)

3.3.1.1
Introduction

Amebiasis, the proper name is pneumonitis, is an infectious disease caused by the protozoan *Entamoeba histolytica*. Worldwide in distribution, it affects 20% of the world population. However, it is most widespread in the tropical countries. The distribution is 0–10% in the northern countries and 5–60% in the tropics. Many of the reported cases in nontropical countries are cases of patients who have visited those areas. This protozoan is harbored initially in the large bowel, causing episodes of acute and chronic diarrhea, along with clinical manifestations ranging from asymptomatic individuals to patients with an acute life-threatening form of the disease. In addition, there are local complications caused by intestinal infection. It may also cause other diseases remotely, via hematogenous processes, such as amebic liver abscess, which is most frequent in extra-intestinal presentation. There are other more atypical complications, such as cerebral or splenic abscess. Major clinical manifestations, including meningoencephalopathy, have also been reported.

3.3.1.2
Epidemiology

Humans are the principal host and reservoir of E. *histolytica*, even though amebic cysts may be found in the large bowel of various animals, including dogs, cats, primates, and rats. Infections tend to be more common in male adults than in children, correlating with a 3:1 ratio. E. *histolytica* is found worldwide from the polar areas to the tropics, and its incidence is inversely proportional to the degree of hygiene habits in a given area. It causes 50–100,000 reported deaths per year and represents the second leading cause of death by a parasitic disease worldwide, primarily in developing countries, where poor habits of hygiene are a common problem.

The propagation of amebiasis is caused by deficiencies in the elementary rules of hygiene, lack of proper sewer systems, and the subsequent contamination of water. The infection is transmitted mainly by carriers who pass cysts directly to other persons (fecal-oral contact) or indirectly, by ingesting cysts of the protozoan E. *histolytica* in polluted food or drinking water.

The risk factors for this infection include poor personal and environmental habits of hygiene, promiscuity, hospitalization in psychiatric institutions, overcrowding, malnutrition, and irrigation with water polluted by feces and the subsequent ingesting of food produced under such conditions. Another important factor is visiting endemic areas. There are population groups particularly prone to having severe forms of the disease, such as children, newborns, pregnant women and women in the postpartum stage, patients under treatment with corticosteroids who are carriers of malign concomitant diseases, and undernourished children and adults.

In the industrialized countries, diagnosed cases generally correspond to travelers who visited endemic areas, or groups of temporary or settled immigrants, as are, for example, the cases in European Mediterranean countries or the south of the United States. Consequently, when evaluating these population groups, amebiasis must be taken into account as a pathology that should be included in our differential diagnosis scheme.

3.3.1.3
Etiology and Pathogenesis

Entamoeba histolytica may exist in two ways, trophozoites (the invasive pathogen form) and cysts (human-infecting form). Trophozoites are not able to become cysts outside the intestine and, thus, they die rapidly outside that environment. A person is infected by ingesting cysts expelled by carriers. Once these cysts are ingested, they pass through the acid environment of the stomach and undergo an ultimate nuclear division. In the intervening time, the cyst has its wall dissolved in the small bowel, and trophozoites are then released. The cysts are then carried along the large bowel, where they feed themselves on bacteria and cells and subsequently adhere to the walls of the colon. In the ileocecal region, they multiply by binary fission and obtain nourishment from the cells of the intestine walls, where phagocytosis takes place. This is the reason why traces of cells, hematic leukocytes are seen in its ectoplasm. The disease–*histolytic*–was therefore named after this phenomenon. Trophozoites have extraordinary motility, due to their rapid emission and uninterrupted contraction as pseudopodia. If they move on through the colon, some of them become round and keep inside a large glycogen vacuole to nourish themselves, thereby forming the so-called pre-cysts. In the recto-sigmoid region and even outside that region, pre-cysts develop a rigid cell wall so that they cease to be mononucleate and become tetranucleate, i.e., they become mature and infecting cysts. Once these cysts are ingested, their nuclei undergo an additional division due to action of the gastric secretions and, as a result, eight trophozoites are released, which will continue the cycle.

The pathogenicity of the invasive amoebae depends on factors such as the ability to adhere to the intestinal walls, the generation of amebic cytolytic and proteolytic effects, and the resistance of this parasite against the defense mechanisms of the host. Pathogen amoebae adhere to the epithelial cell lines Caco-2 and HT-29 through lecithins. The amebic cytolytic activity relies on the function of microfilaments of this parasite, the variety of cysteine-proteinase (the most active among all amebic proteinases), and the ability to keep an acid pH in the endocytic vesicles of the amoeba. Death of intestinal cells occurs up to 20 minutes after amoebae have adhered. Thus, micro-ulcers are initially created that grow in order to produce amebic ulcers, representing the basic anatomic lesion of intestinal amebiasis.

Ulcers exhibit a necrosis that reaches the muscular wall and produces arteriolar thrombosis, thus affecting mucosal irrigation. These effects boost the growth of the ulcer and the detachment of that mucosa. The ulcers can become tissue-penetrating and can burrow into the layers of muscular and serosa tissue and consequently cause peritonitis.

Amoebae reach the liver through portal circulation. In that organ, these are usually destroyed, thus causing only a reactive hepatitis that is not significant. However, due to mechanisms that are not yet well understood, sometimes the amoebae lead to the formation of a hepatic abscess, which is the most frequent manifestation of extra-intestinal amebiasis. The lesion usually has margins that are well defined by a "crown" made of hepatic tissue with lymphocytic and polymorphonuclear infiltration. The content of this abscess is thick and dark, resembling "anchovy paste" and where amoebae are not found. Parasites are found in the margins of this lesion. Amoebae can eventually migrate and affect other organs such as the brain, lungs, and spleen. However, this phenomenon is unusual.

3.3.1.4
Clinical Manifestations

Infected individuals are mostly asymptomatic carriers, with up to 80% of cases corresponding to the commonest type of infection. When in the "carrier status," amoebic individuals do not show symptoms or antibody responses, as this is only a luminal infection. Symptomatic manifestations include:

1. intestinal manifestations that appear after a 7–15-day incubation period with symptoms that can become chronic or acute
2. extra-intestinal disease, and
3. complications.

Chronic Intestinal Manifestations
This is the most frequent clinical manifestation, beginning gradually with mild discomfort, moderate anorexia and asthenia, diffuse abdominal pain, and doughy or semi-liquid evacuations with mucus or blood. The general condition is not strongly affected, nor is there fever. Within 1–2 weeks, symptoms become more intense and apparent, and the number of diarrheic episodes may be up to 4–8 per day in the mildest cases. These symptoms appear as outbreaks and may last for weeks. After a while, they disappear spontaneously. These cycles can be repeated several times during a year.

There are more severe cases, where ulcers tend to spread all through the colon and generally affect the recto-sigmoid area, causing more intense and diffuse abdominal pain, with bloody evacuations that may reach 15–20 per day; there is fever, and the general conditions are affected as patients lose weight and present a decrease in hemoglobin. There is also a high hydro-electrolytic imbalance.

Acute Intestinal Manifestations

Also referred to as fulminant amebic colitis, acute intestinal manifestations appear less frequently and present a very high level of mortality, with a tendency to develop in undernourished individuals, pregnant women, patients under treatment with corticosteroids, and very young individuals. Clinical manifestations begin very rapidly, affecting the individual severely, with 39–40°C fever, intense abdominal colic, profuse diarrhea with tenesmus, and presence of mucus and blood, hypotension, and signs of peritoneal lesions. Hepatomegaly is very frequent, and palpation of the abdomen is very painful. This form of clinical presentation can be associated with the appearance of hepatic abscess. It is usually possible to observe segmentary or total necrosis of the colon, where total colectomy may be necessary; despite good treatment, the condition can cause death. Up to 75% of patients with fulminant colitis are affected by single or multiple colonic perforations, which considerably complicate the prognosis for these patients.

Toxic megacolon is a well documented complication of amebic colitis which is present in 0.5% of cases and is the result of inappropriate treatment with corticosteroids. Patients suffering from toxic megacolon do not respond to drug therapy and thus require surgery.

Ameboma is an amebic granuloma that exhibits a palpable and painful mass which is located outside the liver and appears as an annular lesion, very similar to colon cancer in appearance. Single or multiple, it may exhibit necrosis or edema of the colon mucosa or submucosa and is generally located in the cecum or upper colon. Patients report dysentery and abdominal pain as the main symptoms (see Fig. 2.50). Thus, the presence of ameboma may be confirmed prior to making any surgical decisions. This lesion may, in turn, get worse and present perforations caused by penetrating ulcers, leading to generalized peritonitis or peritonitis that is seldom focused with pericolic abscess formation.

Extra-intestinal Manifestations

The most frequent form of presentation is the hepatic abscess, which is not usually accompanied by an active intestinal disease. However, it may at times appear with colitis. Generally, in the interview, patients do not have a history of previous intestinal amebiasis. Some authors, however, report 50% of cases with such a history.

Abscess may be in the acute form (fewer than 10 days) accompanied by high (39–40 °C) fever and abdominal pain or, in the subacute form, by a considerable loss of weight, vomiting, chills, anorexia, possible jaundice, pain in the right hypochondrium (most frequent symptom) and, depending on the lesion localization, pain in the shoulders, right scapula or, less frequently, in the epigastrium. Hepatomegaly is a common finding, and there can be a nonproductive irritating cough.

Hepatic lesions are produced by lysing that is, in turn, caused by the proteolytic enzymes of *E. histolytica*, primarily hyaluronidase and others, such as cathepsin B proteinase, collagenase, and neutral proteinase. The abscess begins as a small necrotic focus that is formed by the combination of neighboring micro-abscesses that grow as a single lesion. The right lobe is most frequently affected, especially in the posterior segment, due to the predominant irrigation coming from the right colon and due to the larger amount of blood coming from the right branch of the portal system.

In an amebic abscess, necrotic phenomena take precedence over inflammatory phenomena. Three main areas have been identified within an abscess:

1. Central zone, necrotic aspect
2. Middle zone, revealing destruction of parenchyma cells
3. Peripheral zone, where there is still normal hepatic tissue in which amoebae are found.

Complications

The presence of pericardial friction rub, pleural effusion, bloody sputum, or peritonitis is an indication of the appearance of complications caused by draining of the abscess to the pericardium space, pleura, or abdominal cavity. Pleuro-pulmonary amebiasis is the most frequent complication of amebic hepatic abscess. Empyema caused by the rupture and draining of the abscess presents a 15–35% mortality rate. Hepatobronchial fistulae are common. Rupture into the pericardium area is unusual, but is considered a major lesion that becomes apparent in cardiac tamponade and shock, when the rupture is acute. More frequently, the rupture is subacute and is accompanied by fever or abdominal pain, developing into intense thoracic pain and subsequent signs of heart failure.

Peritoneal rupture may occur in 2–7% of cases and, if perforations are abrupt, clinical manifestations are characteristically fatal. Most probably, left lobe abscesses develop to rupture due to their clinical appearance, which is slower.

There are other extra-intestinal manifestations that are less frequent, such as cerebral amebiasis initiating cerebral abscesses. The evolution of this entity is extremely abrupt and, if not treated properly and promptly, develops to death within 12–72 hours.

Genitourinary amebiasis is unusual. There can be dissemination of trophozoites in women to the genitourinary tract through recto-vaginal fistula. Penile amebiasis may occur after anal or vaginal penetration.

Cutaneous amebiasis was previously considered a local complication of colostomy opening or, as an exceptional case, a complication of abscess fistulization into the thoracic wall. Increasing sexual promiscuity has caused this disease to be included in the list of sexually transmitted diseases. Muco-cutaneous lesions commonly have an ulcerous appearance alternating with a condylomatous appearance.

3.3.1.5
Diagnosis

Diagnosis must be supported by an adequate clinical history, physical examination, and para-clinical examinations, such as laboratory tests, X-rays, scintigraphy, computerized axial tomography, magnetic resonance, and ultrasound. Results will depend on localization and presentation of the disease.

Laboratory tests allow the identification of trophozoites or cysts of *E. histolytica* in the feces, positive copro-culture, presence of neutrophilic leukocytosis, positive serology (up to 96%), and an increase in the rate sedimentation of packed red cells in intestinal manifestations. Simple thoracic-abdominal X-rays allow the identification of hepatomegaly and elevation of the hemidiaphragm in cases of hepatic abscess. Scintigraphy allows the identification of areas with the least concentrations of radioisotopes in the liver, but is costly and barely specific. Computerized tomography and magnetic resonance imaging are highly sensitive but have low specificity. Other disadvantages are the use of radiation in the case of tomography, the need to use contrast materials in many cases, and the high cost of equipment and studies, especially in poor or developing countries. Colonoscopy shows the presence of ulcers in the walls of the organ where biopsy samples can be taken.

3.3.1.6
Ultrasound

Ultrasound has proved an excellent method for the diagnosis of hepatic abscess, not only because of its capability to detect lesions, but also because of its particular characteristics such as portability, precision, accessibility, and relative low cost of studies. Using ultrasound, we can calculate the number of lesions, their localization, size, and even the degree of liquefaction. Most hepatic abscesses have a pyogenic origin (88%); those with an amebic or fungal origin are less frequent, at 10% and 2%, respectively. All types of abscesses, regardless of their etiology, can be detected using ultrasound. However, in up to 50% of cases it is not possible to determine the etiologic origin. This method is also useful in the detection of residual lesions.

3.3.1.7
Hepatic Abscesses

It is worth mentioning that, in the initial phases, amoebic hepatic abscesses may not be detectable and thus ultrasound findings look absolutely normal, which is not unusual in our clinical practice (Fig. 3.41a). When lesions become visible to ultrasound, they generally have a round or oval shape in up to 82% of patients, and present fine echoes in the core in 56% of cases (unlike pyogenic abscesses, where these characteristics may reach 60% and 36%, respectively). Amebic abscesses are less echogenic than hepatic parenchyma. Amebic abscesses are mostly localized in the periphery of the right lobe and adjacent to the hepatic capsule. Contiguity with the diaphragm can also be observed. Variable in size, rare cases of extremely large proportions have been reported, straddling the upper abdomen and the pelvis. Amebic hepatic abscesses are generally detected as a single occurrence, but they can also appear as multiple instances, usually with poorly defined walls. It has a hypoechoic, cystic (Fig. 3.41c), or complicated-cyst image (depending on the degree of liquefaction) and presents posterior acoustic enhancement with variable intensity in 70–80% of cases (Figs. 3.41, 3.42). In our experience, Doppler ultrasound shows peripheral flow with a mild signal intensity and unspecific in nature (Fig. 3.43).

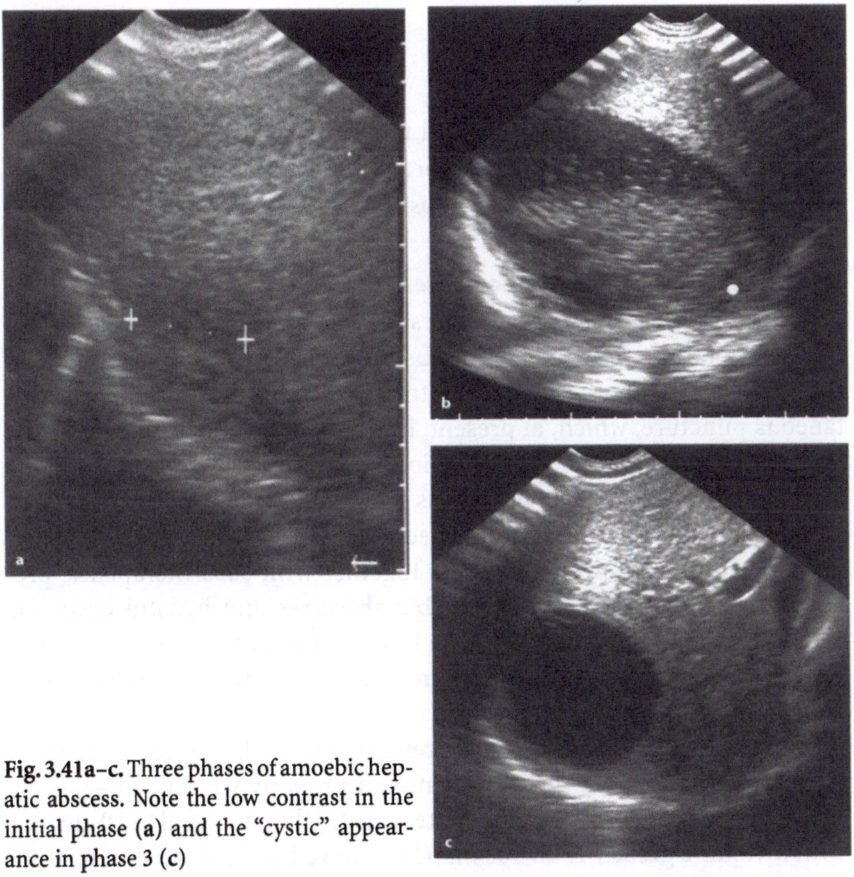

Fig. 3.41a–c. Three phases of amoebic hepatic abscess. Note the low contrast in the initial phase (**a**) and the "cystic" appearance in phase 3 (**c**)

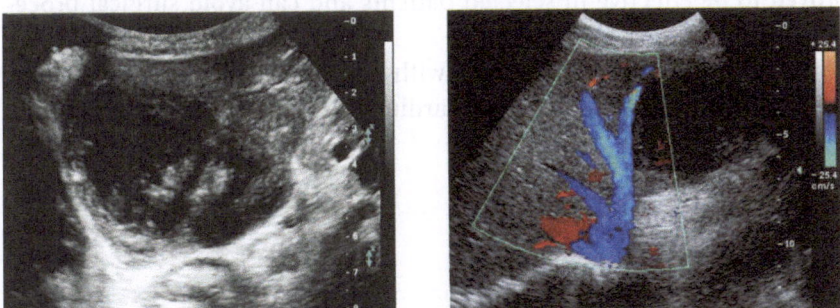

Fig. 3.42. Huge amoebic abscess in the left lobe with an irregular echo pattern

Fig. 3.43. Amoebic liver abscess: Note the CD-signals in the periphery of the abscess

3.3.1.8
Differential Diagnosis

The above sonographic findings call for differential diagnosis from pyogenic abscesses, hemorrhagic cysts, or subsequently abscessing hematomas and hepatic tumors with inner necrosis.

Treatment of Amoebic Hepatic Abscess

Advanced medical treatment restores to health the majority of individuals suffering from amebic hepatic abscess. However, extensive lesions or refractory cases to anti-amoebic treatment may require draining by percutaneous puncture, which, at present, is a safe (and sometimes necessary) procedure with negligible complications.

Ultrasound is a convenient means for establishing orientation in percutaneous puncture. Giorgi published a study where results from 16,648 3D-assisted biopsies were reviewed, together with 3035 therapeutic procedures, both for pyogenic or amebic abscesses and hydatid cysts and ablations using radiofrequency. The level of mortality in these cases was 0.6%. There were neither deaths nor major complications after draining of hepatic abscesses.

Patients requiring percutaneous puncture of their abscesses are those who do not respond to medical treatment properly within a 48–72-hour period, present lesions with a diameter greater than or equal to 10 cm, and with a volume greater than 300 ml. Cases have been reported of patients in which the rupture of abscesses was resolved by placement of a catheter for percutaneous drainage. The combination of medical treatment with metronidazole and percutaneous drainage with or without catheters has proved to be effective in selected patients and can avoid surgical procedures.

Surgery is reserved for patients with important complications such as empyema, drainage into the pericardium, and major drainage into the peritoneal cavity.

3.3.1.9
Post-Treatment Evolution

The healing process is evidenced by the progressive reduction of abscess size. The cavity may last for weeks or months after medical treatment has been completed, with an average of seven months. Total recovery may require up to two years. A small group of patients may remain with residual hepatic cysts or focal areas with increased or decreased echogenicity.

3.3.2
Trypanosomiasis

3.3.2.1
American Trypanosomiasis (Chagas' Disease)
(by Alfonso J.G. Barbato, Nathan Herszkowicz, Waldir Salvi, Nestor de Barros, Giovanni G. Cerri)

Introduction
Chagas' disease was first described by a Brazilian doctor named Carlos Chagas in 1909. This disease is confined to the American continent, spreading from the south of the United States to Argentina, with about 15 to 20 million infected people, at least 4 to 6 million of them in Brazil. It is an important public health problem because its manifestations affect young adults, frequently between the second and fourth decades.

This disease is usually rural, caused by *Trypanosoma cruzi*, transmitted through fecal material produced by *Triatoma* bugs (insects that live in the walls of poor houses) . The fecal material is inoculated around the bite or by ocular and oral mucosa, and by blood transfusion infrequently. Insect eradication, improvement of social conditions, better housing, and control of blood donors reduce the incidence of the disease, the super-infections, and the re-infections, probably decreasing the gravity of the manifestations of the disease and raising the age of patients at the onset of the infection.

The local infection by *T. cruzi* can start immunological responses and inflammatory reactions that can affect the local microcirculation, with consequent fibrosis and parasympathetic denervation.

Neurological, cardiac, and digestive abnormalities are observed. According to the presentation, the disease can be divided into three phases based on clinical manifestations as follows:

Acute
seldom observed, presents cutaneous, neurologic, gastric, and cardiac involvement; abdominal adenomegaly and fever are also present. In chronic or indeterminate phases, an atypical manifestation of "re-acuteness" is observed in immunodepressed patients, e.g., transplant recipients or patients with AIDS.

Undetermined

asymptomatic with pathologic laboratory findings. The majority of patients are in this phase. The disease is detected by serology in epidemiological screening examinations and in blood donors. A progressive pattern is not yet established to define which and how many patients are going to develop the chronic phase. Although asymptomatic, probably most of these patients have minor digestive and cardiac morphological and functional manifestations. These patients, when submitted to different imaging examinations, usually show abnormalities in more than one of these parameters.

Chronic

symptomatic, with significant clinical, cardiac, and digestive manifestations. Different strains of *T. cruzi* can affect one organ more than others, and digestive manifestations are usually found only in Brazil, where cardiac and digestive involvement in the same patient is common.

Cardiac Manifestations

The cardiac manifestations are caused by the cardiomyopathy and its consequences. Chronic segmental cardiomyopathy and fibrotic areas are the most common alteration with morphological and functional cardiac involvement. The right ventricle frequently is involved, which differs from other cardiomyopathies; apical aneurysms (uncommon localization in others cardiomyopathies) are also frequent. Arrhythmia and thrombus (responsible for systemic embolism) are common causes of premature death in the chronic phase.

Echocardiography

In the acute phase, two-dimensional echocardiography shows a decrease in cardiac performance, usually found in myocarditis and pericardial effusion, which is quite common.

The echocardiographic examination in the undetermined phase usually is normal, but may show:

(a) minor involvement, with a dilated, adapted phase in which we observe an enlargement of the heart with normal motility; the systolic volume is increased but the ventricular function is preserved
(b) segmental lesion of the apical myocardium (Fig. 3.44a,b), especially in the postero-inferior wall with preserved ventricular septum and slight

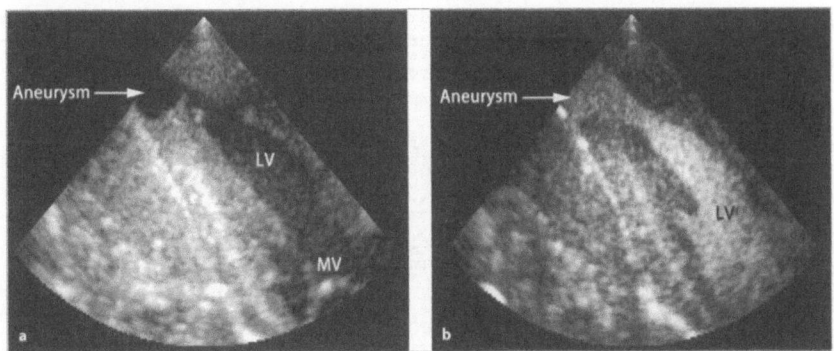

Fig. 3.44a,b. Apical aneurysm in the left ventricle, without a thrombus (**a**). Opacification of the apical aneurysm using microbubbles (**b**). Transesophageal echocardiogram, long axis

hypokinesis. These signs help to differentiate this cardiomyopathy from others

(c) alteration of the myocardial contraction with the use of isoproterenol and isotonic effort maneuvers (emphasizing the importance of a complete color Doppler echocardiographic examination).

Tissue Doppler is useful in detecting the segmental lesions and regional systolic alterations (Fig. 3.45).

In the chronic phase, the findings basically reflect cardiac dilatation and compromise of the cardiac function. The two-dimensional echocardiographic examination can detect:

(a) dilatation and diffuse myocardial lesion (characterizing the cardiomyopathy), with increased relationship between volume/mass rate (Fig. 3.46),

(b) left ventricular systolic and diastolic volume enlargement,

(c) septal and postero-inferior wall hypokinesis,

(d) segmental hypokinesis of the posterior wall of the left ventricle,

(e) diffuse hypokinetic pattern that can be observed in up to 25% of cases,

(f) decrease in ventricular function, with reduction of the ejection.

(These abnormalities can occur together.)

This method may also detect frequent complications of the chronic phase represented by apical aneurysms (pathognomonic of this disease) and mural thrombi (Fig. 3.47).

Doppler and color-Doppler echocardiography may detect mitral regurgitation due to left ventricular enlargement and dysfunction of papillary

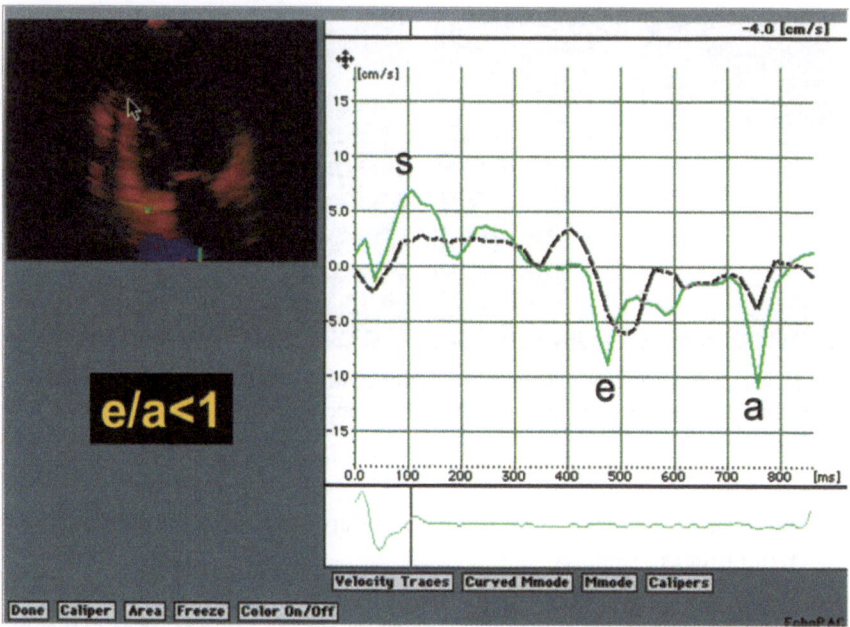

Fig. 3.45. Chagas' disease in undetermined phase with diastolic dysfunction. Two-dimensional echocardiogram. The apical view shows tissue Doppler of the left ventricle

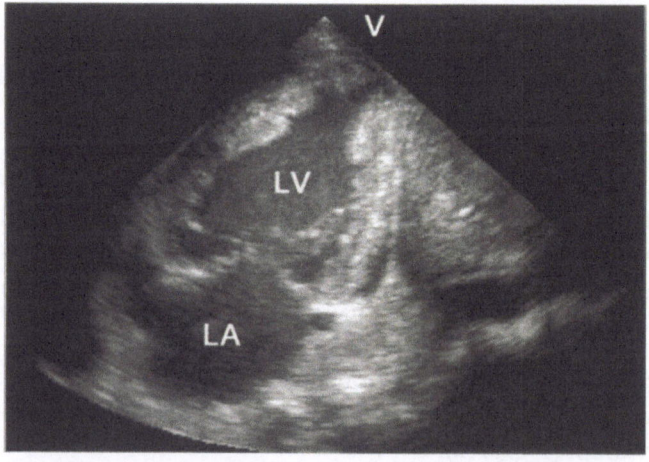

Fig. 3.46. Enlargement of the left ventricle and a diffuse hypokinetic pattern in Chagas' disease. Two-dimensional echocardiogram, apical view, two chambers

Fig. 3.47. Biventricular volume enlargement and mural thrombus in the right ventricle. Two-dimensional echocardiogram, apical view, four chambers

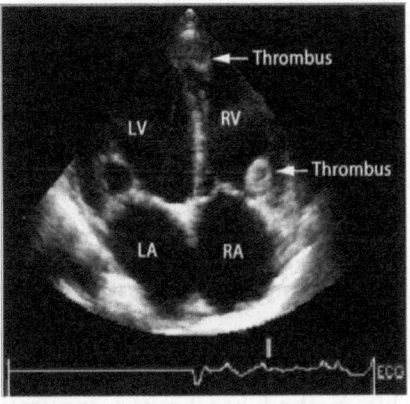

muscles and valve dilatation and low ventricular flow, typical of diffuse ventricular disease.

Digestive Manifestations
In the acute phase, the digestive manifestations are rarely seen and are not clinically important. Hepatosplenomegaly and adenomegaly are observed.

In the undetermined and chronic phases, the digestive disease is produced by minor to accentuated reduction of the myoenteric plexus and is manifested by variable degree of motor dysfunction and visceromegaly (called mega), findings that are observed in almost all hollow viscera. The motor dysfunction presents mainly as inability to coordinate the opening of the hypertrophied sphincter functioning as a barrier to peristaltic wave.

Undetermined Phase The patient is usually asymptomatic, but esophageal manometry with pentagastrin or cholinergic stimulation may disclose abnormality, represented by high pressure of the inferior esophageal sphincter in almost all patients.

Chronic Phase The most prominent findings are found in this phase.

The esophagus is the organ most commonly affected, followed by the colon. Association with carcinomas usually of the inferior third of the esophagus (up to 3% of patients with large mega-esophagus) is observed.

The pyloric dysfunction is present in up to 22% of patients with intermediate or advanced stage mega-esophagus, and is diagnosed if gastric emptying does not happen in more than two hours. The duodenal dysfunction is present in up to 1.5% of patients with intermediate or advanced stage mega-esophagus.

Mega-gallbladder is infrequent, but vesicular calculus is present in up to 7% of the patients with mega-esophagus, and can be found in patients with cardiac manifestations.

It is important to emphasize that the alterations of the digestive organs seldom occur in isolation, and it is common that patients with mega-esophagus also present with megacolon and cardiomyopathy.

Ultrasound

This method has limited application in the study of digestive manifestations. Abdominal ultrasound shows hepatosplenomegaly and adenomegaly in the rarely observed acute phase. Ultrasound is the method of choice in detecting the infrequent mega-gallbladder and the presence of vesicular calculus. Occasionally in the chronic phase, ultrasound shows in longitudinal view of the superior abdomen, behind the liver and above the diaphragm, the distal portion of the large mega-esophagus tapered at the esophagogastric transition, with strong echoes inside.

Although well established radiologically, ultrasonographic evaluation of gastric emptying delay is still an subject of experimental research and can be diagnosed by the absence of significant change in antral diameters of orthostatic right paramedian views two hours after gastric filling with 300 ml (creamy) food introduced by nasal-gastric tube. The place of endoscopic ultrasound in staging the carcinoma associated with mega-esophagus in Chagas' disease is not yet established.

In conclusion, ultrasound, mainly echocardiography, is useful in the diagnoses and morphological evaluation, but mainly in the functional evaluation of Chagas cardiomyopathy and its complications as a noninvasive method. This method is also useful in diagnosing gall bladder manifestation.

3.3.2.2
African Trypanosomiasis, Sleeping Sickness
(by Harald Th. Lutz)

Introduction

African Trypanosomiasis is limited to equatorial Africa. In 1901, *Trypanosoma brucei rhodesiense* and *Trypanosoma brucei gambiense* were identified as the pathogenic organism causing this protozoan disease. The parasites are transmitted by the painful bites of the tsetse fly. These two parasites are morphologically identical, but *T. rhodesiense* causes a more severe disease in East Africa, whereas *T. gambiense* causes a more chronic and mild disease in the western part of Africa, which, untreated, may involve the CNS after a period of months.

In contrast to Chagas' disease, the parasites cannot be demonstrated in the histological tissue specimen.

Pathology
The bite of an infected fly causes a local reaction and a local lymphadenitis. With hematogenic dissemination, the lymph nodes, spleen, heart, and especially the CNS then become involved. In the beginning stage of the CNS disease, meningitis develops, followed by encephalitis in the late stage.

Ultrasonography
In the acute stage, it is possible to demonstrate enlarged lymph nodes, splenomegaly, and fluid in various body cavities. All of these findings are not specific for the disease.

Furthermore, the symptoms of pancarditis may be demonstrated by echocardiography, as described in detail in section 3.3.2.1. In the chronic stage, the fibrosis of the endocardium can be detected with echocardiography.

In contrast to Chagas' disease, the CNS rather than the heart is the clinically important manifestation of African trypanosomiasis. Ultrasound is of minor importance in this protozoan disease.

3.3.3
Ascariasis
(by Leandro J. Fernandez)

3.3.3.1
Overview

Helminthes or worms are particularly notorious metazoans among infectious agents, owing to their size, prevalence, complexity of their vital cycles, and their migrations within the host. Other outstanding characteristics include their ability to produce eosinophilia as well as their inability to directly replicate inside humans. Unlike fungi, viruses, bacteria, and other parasites, which are only visible by microscopy, all helminths are visible with the naked eye, with their length varying from 2 to 10,000 mm. Nematodes or round worms exhibit a lengthened shape with a circular section and bilateral symmetry. These organisms have a gastrointestinal tract and sexual dimorphism. With over 500,000 species, most of them lead a free life and only a few are parasites in humans, thereby producing major diseases. Depending on their biology and growth cycles, they fall into two categories of nematodes, both of them harmful to humans: intestinal nematodes and titrated nematodes.

Ascaris lumbricoides is a nematode which commonly infects humans and is responsible for the most frequent intestinal helminthiasis. Its prevalence is very high in tropical and subtropical regions where hygiene conditions are unfavorable. Consequently, they represent a major public health problem in many poor or developing countries.

3.3.3.2
Epidemiology

Ascariasis is a disease caused by the presence of *A. lumbricoides* in the upper parts of the small bowel. *A. lumbricoides* is the largest intestinal nematode. With a worldwide prevalence, it is estimated that more than 1000 million individuals are carriers, especially in the tropics, and up to 25% of this population suffers from ascariasis. Several studies have reported this high prevalence, especially in the school population from many developing countries, with values varying from 12% to 90%. The prevalence of ascariasis is directly associated with poor hygiene conditions and very low economic and sociocultural levels. The degree of incidence is exacerbated by malnutrition, the parasitic load, and the peculiar parasite biology.

The infection appears in individuals of all ages but tends to be more widespread in preschool and early school children. Its incidence is similar for both sexes and, in the United States, for instance, it mainly affects the black population of the South East of the country, in a 3:1 correlation with respect to the white population. Cases of polyparasitosis cohabitating with *A. lumbricoides*, *Trichuris trichura*, *Strongyloides stercoralis*, and *Ancylostoma duodenale* are fairly common.

3.3.3.3
Etiology and Pathogenesis

A. lumbricoides is a cylinder-shaped worm which, in its adult stage, reaches 20–40 cm in length and is 5 mm thick. This organism is motile and has a strong muscular mass; its color is white, pink, or reddish-yellow, and it inhabits the small bowel, especially the jejunum and the ileum, but without adhering to the walls. It remains in the intestinal space, because of its characteristic muscular tone. Its half-life is 1–2 years, and each female parasite produces some 200,000 eggs per day. The fertile eggs are oval-shaped and very resistant to severe environmental conditions: they can survive up to 2 years at a temperature of 5–10 °C, or 3 months in the absence of oxygen, and they are able to endure desiccation for up to 2–3 weeks at a temperature of 22 °C. In wet, soft and sandy soil, they keep viable for up to 6 years and are able to tolerate the freezing temperatures of the winter. When in wet soil, larvae develop inside of the eggs within a 2–3-week period, particularly if this soil is clayey, maintains a cool temperature, and remains under shadow. Contagion takes place by carrying cysts from the hands to the mouth, and by ingesting contaminated water or food (especially vegetables that have been watered using egg-contaminated water or food from crops fertilized with human feces). Once embryonate eggs are ingested, they make it to the digestive tract and have their coats dissolved by the digestive juices and, as a result, larvae are released. These forms penetrate the intestinal wall and move on through the portal circulation to reach the lungs within a 7-day period, where they penetrate the alveoli, ascend through the trachea and are swallowed to return to the digestive tract. A period of 2 months is required for larvae to become gravida and for the first eggs to appear in the feces. Anatomopathological changes produced by this parasite are in turn the result of migrations and the action of parasitic load.

3.3.3.4
Clinical Presentation

Ascariasis has two presentation forms; pulmonary and intestinal. Pulmonary ascariasis is the result of the migration of larvae and typically produces 37.5–40 °C fever, paroxysmal cough, hemoptysis, retrosternal discomfort, dyspnea, chills, and pulmonary sibilants (Löffler syndrome). Pulmonary symptoms are associated with pulmonary infiltration and marked eosinophilia as well as urticaria-like reactions in 15% of cases, or are associated with angioneurotic edema, especially in those patients with previous sensitization. Fortunately, only a small number of patients suffer from this presentation compared to the huge number of patients affected by ascariasis.

Löffler syndrome typically lasts one week. Tracheobronchitis symptoms and rapidly changing pulmonary infiltrates, followed by important peripheral eosinophilia, are common features. Basically a syndrome that appears mostly in adults, IgE alterations and eosinophilia shows that this disease is the result of hypersensitivity reactions. In endemic areas where ascariasis infection is seasonal, seasonal pneumonitis has been described.

Abdominal manifestations are dependent on the amount of parasites residing in the digestive tract and, typically, patients are asymptomatic. The first indication of parasitosis frequently consists of the emergence of worms through the mouth, nose, or rectum. When the parasite load is moderate, nonspecific digestive alterations may appear, such as abdominal colic pain, hyporexia, nausea, vomiting, and even intestinal malabsorption. It is worth mentioning that, at this stage, eosinophilia decreases and may even disappear. In cases of high parasite load, especially in children, vermes pack together within the small bowel to produce pseudo-obstruction, intestinal obstruction, intussusceptions, or volvulus, a fairly common situation in the least developed countries owing in turn to the poor social and economic (and therefore deficient nutritional) conditions. These abdominal manifestations are life-threatening if not treated properly.

Some patients with helminthes-related hypersensitivity reactions may develop urticaria, dyspnoea, and bronchial asthma. Other individuals may develop epileptic seizures or feverish saccade and irritability due to the action of endotoxins present in adult *Ascaris*. These clinical manifestations are referred to as "ascaridian encephalopathy."

There are other manifestations which we shall refer to as ascariasis complications. As helminthes are remarkably motile, they are able to migrate to the choledochus, where they can initiate a partial or total obstruction. They can also reach the gall bladder, Wirsung's duct, and the cecal appendix. These presentation forms are usually found in children and patients with different degrees of malnutrition. The movements cause cholecystitis and pancreatitis. Being able to cause the formation of pyogenic abscesses, *Ascaris* in hepatic parenchyma has been less frequently described in the literature.

There are also even more atypical complications, such as perforation of the intestinal wall and the transfer of vermes through the intestinal sutures.

3.3.3.5
Diagnosis

Diagnosis is made by establishing the presence of parasites in feces, vomiting, and spontaneous emergence of worms through body orifices, or by detecting the presence of cysts in the patient's feces, which generally occurs as of the second month after contagion. The presence of larvae in the sputum and gastric aspirate is an unusual finding, if samples coincide with a titrated migration. Abdominal X-rays allow the observation of intestinal nematodes and, if a barium contrast study is performed, the occurrence of parasites is clearly highlighted, including the intestinal tract. Magnetic resonance imaging is also a useful method to diagnose the parasite, since it allows a cholangiographic visualization and defines the presence of nematodes and their structure. Anti-*Ascaris* IgG4 antibodies have been determined in India with good results. High levels of these serum antibodies are seen in patients with acute infection who returned to normal values after 6 months of treatment. Santra suggested that this method be used as a diagnostic test for epidemiological studies. It is also known that elevation of serum levels of IgE occurs because of the antigenic components of *Ascaris*. This elevation has been associated with hypersensitivity processes in atopic patients.

Ultrasound is an excellent technique that allows the observation of these parasites with the added advantages that it is safe and inexpensive, has no side effects, and is available even in rural areas.

3.3.3.6
Sonographic Findings

It is possible, by ultrasound, to locate parasites within the anatomic areas already mentioned, such as the small bowel, the biliary tract, the gall bladder, and even the hepatic parenchyma, although this presentation is unusual. In some patients, ingesting water prior to the ultrasound examination generates an acoustic window that allows a better visualization of this parasite in the intestine. *A. lumbricoides* is seen in the longitudinal section as a lengthened echogenic structure, which usually does not produce any acoustic back shadow (unless the parasite has died and

Fig. 3.48. Ascariasis. Transverse scan through the liver and the hilus, showing worms in longitudinal and cross-section

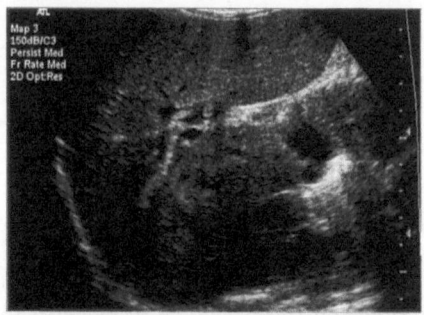

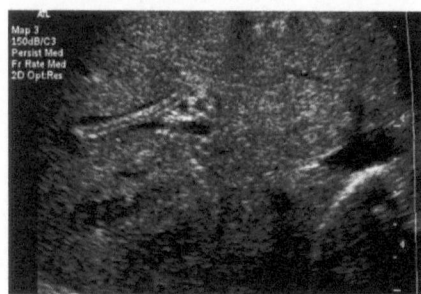

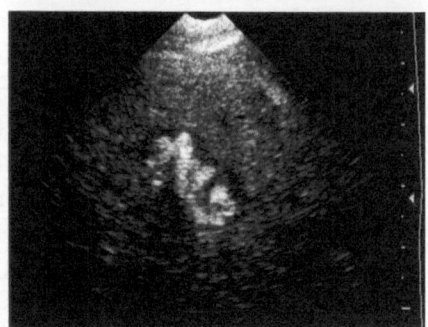

Fig. 3.49. Ascarids in the intrahepatic bile ducts

Fig. 3.50. Ascariasis: roundworms "within" the liver

has subsequently calcified). Inside this organism, a hypoechoic image is seen that encompasses the complete structure of the helminthes, i.e., its gastrointestinal tract. Three or four interfaces are seen that are related with the anterior and posterior walls and the gastrointestinal tract; in the cross-section, it is possible to see a rounded image that resembles a dial (Fig. 3.48). If the vermis is alive, serpent-like movements can be seen in the echogenic image.

When ascarides are located in the gall bladder, they can be seen both extended and bent and, if calcified, they can be mistaken for lithiasis. Occasionally, we have seen them adhered to the gall bladder wall. If found in the biliary tract, especially in the choledochus, one or several worms can be seen which may cause duct obstruction. We have seen ascarides that migrated to the hepatic parenchyma, causing abscesses, but only in undernourished children. Regardless of their location, the vermis maintains the echogenic features already described (Figs. 3.49–3.52).

Fig. 3.51. Worm demonstrated in the liver parenchyma

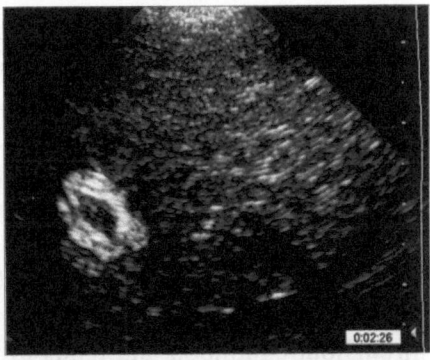

Fig. 3.52. Multiple ascarids in the common bile ducts

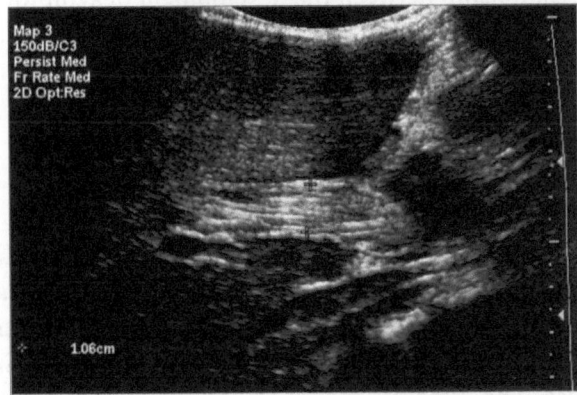

Endoscopic ultrasound has also been used to visualize ascarides, because of its high sensitivity (92%) in the assessment of biliary tract.

3.3.4
Bancroftian Filariasis
(by Gerusa Dreyer, Joaquim Noroes, Fernando Amaral)

3.3.4.1
Epidemiology / Clinical Presentation

Bancroftian filariasis is a vector-borne infection and an important public health problem in tropical and subtropical areas of the world. It persists as a major cause of clinical morbidity and a significant impediment to socioeconomic development in Asia, Africa, and the Western Pacific as well as in certain regions of the Americas. An estimated 100 million persons are infected with *Wuchereria bancrofti*, and overall about 40 million have chronic forms of the disease. The clinical presentation of the disease caused by the adult stage of the parasite stage includes acute filarial lymphangitis (provoked by the death of the adult worm) and chronic manifestations such as subclinical or clinical lymphangiectasia, lymphadenopathy, lymphedema, hydrocele, chylocele, and chyluria (and hematochyluria). The main manifestations caused by microfilariae are tropical pulmonary eosinophilia (TPE) and hematuria.

The chronic sequelae of filarial infection may not become evident until later in life. In contrast, the prevalence of microfilaremia increases throughout childhood and tends to plateau soon after adolescence. The relationship between the development of symptoms and the course of the infection, however, is not completely understood. This is due, largely, to the lack of an experimental model.

3.3.4.2
Pathogenesis

Despite more than a century of scientific study, the pathogenesis of lymphatic damage in filariasis is incompletely understood. It is increasingly recognized, however, that lymphatic vessel dilatation is the central lesion in the development of chronic filarial morbidity in filariasis-endemic areas. The dynamic model of lymphatic filarial disease that we proposed has two basic tenets. Given a sufficient duration of infection, all persons harboring adult worms develop, at least, localized lymphangiectasia in the vicinity of worm nests, which is not caused by mechanical obstruction of the lymphatic vessel but by some other as yet unidentified process. This primordial filaria-induced lymphatic abnormality remains subclinical in the majority of patients with bancroftian filariasis. However, lymphangiectasia constitutes a major risk factor for the development of chronic lymphatic disease, because it can cause lymphatic dysfunction. On the other hand, the lymphatic system has enormous reserve capacity to drain extravasated fluid and solutes from extracellular spaces efficiently under a variety of basal and stress conditions: minor insults to the system rarely cause persistent clinical disease. It is therefore proposed that clinical syndromes of chronic lymphatic disease ordinarily do not develop in bancroftian filariasis unless at least one other factor compounds filaria-induced lymphangiectasia and thereby overwhelms the compensatory capabilities of the lymphatic system. The second concept embedded in the model is the distinction between the pathogenesis of chronic hydroceles, chyloceles, and chyluria with chronic lymphedema. Worms alone are sufficient to cause filarial hydroceles, provided some compounding factor compromises lymphatic drainage. In contrast, chronic lymphedema develops only when the lymphatic system is damaged by two factors acting in concert: these are lymphatic dysfunction and secondary bacterial infections. Recurrent secondary bacterial infections also promote the progression of simple lymphedema to elephantiasis. In both instances, bacterial infections can be clearly identified as essential cofactors.

3.3.4.3
Background

Ultrasound is increasingly used for diagnosis and clinical studies of parasitic diseases such as schistosomiasis and echinococcosis, and recently it has been shown to be a powerful tool for the study of bancroftian filariasis. In 1994, we first reported using ultrasound to visualize adult *W. bancrofti* in the scrotal area of infected men. We described a continuous, distinctive, and specific pattern of worm movement called the "filaria dance sign" (FDS). When patients who exhibited this sign were taken to surgery, the intrascrotal lymphatic vessels that were surgically removed were dilated and tortuous with "nests" of adult *W. bancrofti* which confirmed the ultrasound images. The location of the adult worm nests within the lymphatic vessels remains remarkably stable with time, allowing a maximum level of reproducibility. Extensive clinical and surgical experience has confirmed these initial findings, and ultrasound examinations of men from nonendemic areas have failed to detect the FDS. In adult men, ultrasound has been successfully used to assess, *in vivo*, the adulticidal efficacy of antifilarial drugs, describe preclinical abnormalities in the lymphatic vessels, identify amicrofilaremic adult worm carriers, identify living adult worms in patients with tropical pulmonary eosinophilia; and identify the FDS in children and in the female breast. Recently, ultrasound also was shown to be suitable for detecting living worms in lymph nodes. The FDS has subsequently been reported in India, Egypt, Haiti, the Dominican Republic, Papua New Guinea, Tanzania, and Ghana. Recent studies indicate that dilatation of the lymphatic vessel occurs not only at the site of the adult worm nest, but also more diffusely, in the general vicinity of the worm. Further, dilatation is exceedingly heterogeneous within a given segment of lymphatic vessel; sections of almost normal vessel are interspersed with areas of massive lymphangiectasia. A high degree of lymphatic vessel dilation variability is observed among individuals, and even among different nests within the same individual. The lymphatic vessel dilatation continues to progress even after treatment with currently recommended antifilarial drugs, when, as is often the case, these drugs do not kill all of the living adult *W. bancrofti.*

3.3.4.4
Examination Technique

The purpose of this chapter is to describe the ultrasonographic findings in patients with lymphangiectasia, whether or not they harbor living *W. bancrofti* adult worms in dilated lymphatic vessels and lymph nodes. The chronic forms of morbidity, such as hydrocele and lymphedema, are not discussed here.
Preparation is not required.

Probes
Depending on the purpose, the 3.5, 5.0 (linear array is preferable), 7.5, or the new higher frequency probes such as 14 MHz can be used. M-mode and pulsed Doppler improve accuracy of FDS identification in very small lymphatics. For screening purposes, including screening for suspected lymphangiectasia, a 3.5-MHz probe can be used as a rapid public health tool to monitor filariasis control programs, or even for individual diagnosis, depending on the degree of lymphatic vessel dilation (see pitfalls below).

Anatomic Sites
Routinely the lymphatics vessels of the scrotum (both the skin and intrascrotal) and inguinal cord, the main superficial dilated lymphatic vessels of the legs, arms, and breast, and the superficial lymph nodes can be examined. Examination is done with the patient in the supine position; if needed, for example, women with large breasts may turn 45 degrees to the left or to the right side.

- Scrotal area: The patient should lift the scrotal sac and cross the legs in order to find the best position to screen the entire target area. The examination is initiated with a longitudinal scan from the external side to the midline of each hemiscrotum, and from the top of the scrotal spermatic cord to the bottom of the hemiscrotum contents. A transverse scan is then performed, following the sequence as above. The retrotesticular area should be carefully scanned.

- Superficial lymphatics: The probe should follow the main lymphatic vessel route of the limbs (as known from early studies by lymphangiography and, more recently, by lymphoscintigraphy) and breasts. The examination should be done with a longitudinal and transverse scan.
- Lymph nodes: Any enlarged lymph node on physical examination should be scanned, as is done routinely for any disease.

3.3.4.5
Ultrasound Findings

B-mode ultrasonography shows dilated and tortuous tubular structures (especially in the larger lymphatics), most of the time with anechoic background and no flow (Fig. 3.53), with or without echogenic points and linear short segments in the lumen (Fig. 3.54). The real-time examination reveals peculiar, active, random-appearing movements of those echogenic structures; that is, the filaria dance sign. The movements are different from the well-recognized turbulence of arterial or venous flow. M-mode documents the predominantly transverse movements seen in real time (Fig. 3.55). In pulsed Doppler, the spectrum shows an alleatory pattern of spikes (Fig. 3.56). In color Doppler, a mixture of colors is observed near the mobile echoes and does not help in diagnosing the FDS.

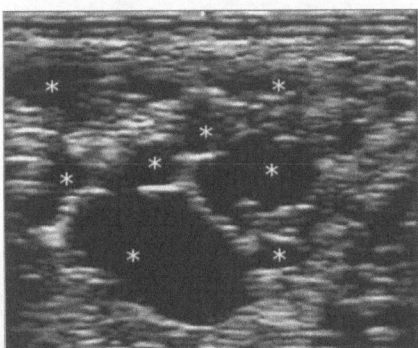

Fig. 3.53. Brazilian 27-year-old male. Spermatic cord ultrasound image in B-mode with 7.5-MHz probe showing cystic-like anechoic structures (*). This finding represents a typical appearance of diffuse lymphangiectasia caused by *W. bancrofti* adult worms

Fig. 3.54. Brazilian 30-year-old male. Ultrasound B-mode with 7.5 MHz showing the testis (**), dilated lymphatic vessel (*) containing transversal hyperechogenic segments of the adult worms *W. bancrofti* (*arrows*) which in real-time examination is called filaria dance sign (FDS) because of their continuous and active movement

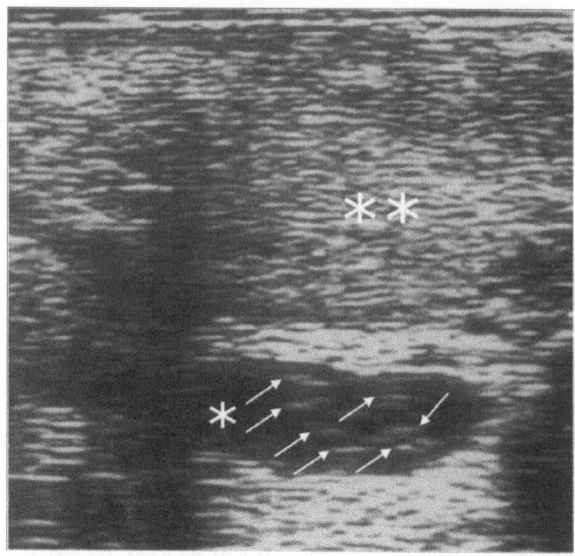

Fig. 3.55. Brazilian 28-year-old male, microfilaria carrier. In B-mode (left side) the testis is seen (**) along with dilated lymphatic vessel (*) containing hyperechogenic linear structures representing the *W. bancrofti* adult worms (*arrows*) with 7.5-MHz probe. The graphic representation of the adult worm movement is seen on M-mode (*right*)

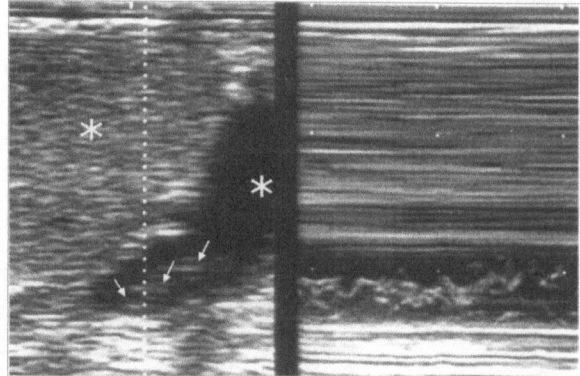

Fig. 3.56. Brazilian 31-year-old male amicrofilaremic adult worm carrier. Pulsed Doppler pattern of FDS (*bottom*) in a small retrotesticular lymphatic vessel (*arrow*)

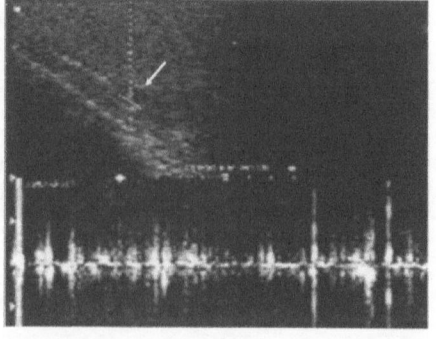

3.3.4.6
Differential Diagnosis

The findings described for the identification of the FDS are very distinctive; however, in some instances, venous blood flow may be confused with the FDS in small vessels. Longer observation in a given site may be needed in order to distinguish between these different patterns of movement. In examination of the intrascrotal area, the Valsalva maneuver may help in the differential diagnosis. Additionally, M-mode is useful to differentiate flow from the worm movement. Ultimately, pulsed Doppler is the ideal way to differentiate blood flow from worm movement. Giant lymphangiectasia may be misdiagnosed as hydrocele. In this case, it is necessary to wait some time to see whether or not adult worms are present. If they do not appear on the screen, it is usually not possible to differentiate giant lymphangiectasia from septate hydrocele by ultrasound.

3.3.4.7
Pitfalls

Thus far, it is not possible to predict by the ultrasound image the number of worms or to determine whether both sexes are present in a given nest. Ultrasound is not suitable for diagnosis of dead worms. Disappearance of the FDS after diethylcarbamazine (DEC) treatment must be confirmed by palpation of a nodule in the location where the worms were seen previously. In the absence of fibrosis or calcification, detection of a filarial granuloma may be difficult, because its echogenicity may be very similar to that of the surrounding tissue. On the other hand, a suspected image of dead worms can be seen in recent granulomas as hyperechogenic lines on a hypoechoic background. Large hydroceles compress the lymphatic vessels, making it difficult (or impossible, in most cases) to visualize the FDS.

Most ultrasound studies of bancroftian filariasis have used 7.5-MHz transducers, which provide good resolution of the superficial and dilated lymphatic vessels harboring living worms. However, the need for a 7.5-MHz transducer greatly limits the use of ultrasound for diagnosis and study of lymphatic filariasis in remote places. We have compared the performance of ultrasound with 3.5- and 7.5-MHz transducers in detecting the FDS in the scrotal area of infected men. Our study indicated that a 3.5-MHz probe can also be used to detect the FDS of *W. bancrofti* (and lymphangiectasia shown in Fig. 3.57) with a relatively high sensitivity (79% of adult worm

Fig. 3.57. Brazilian25-year-old male. Ultrasound of scrotal contents in B-
mode with 3.5-MHz probe showing anechoic cyst-like structures (*arrows*) corresponding to large lymphangiectasias in
an infected patient with *W. bancrofti*. The
FDS (not clear on this image) was seen
in a less dilated lymphatic (*small arrow*).
No hydrocele was present

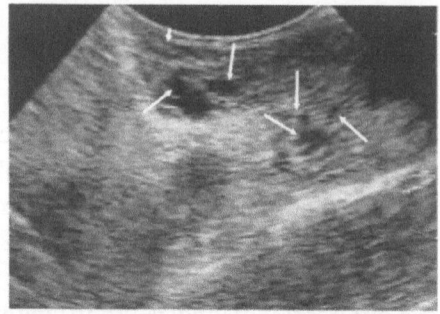

nests and 85% of infected men) and specificity (100%). Detection of the
FDS with the 3.5-MHz transducer was unreliable when the lymphatic vessel
diameter was less than 2.7 mm. Thus, for practical purposes, the limit of
detection for the 3.5-MHz probe was reached at a vessel diameter of 2.7 mm.
For the 7.5-MHz probe, the limit of detection appears to be at a vessel
diameter of approximately 1 mm. Thus, when maximum resolution of the
ultrasound image is required, such as in studies of drug efficacy, the 7.5-
MHz transducer should continue to be used, in this case, always combined
with physical examination.

3.3.4.8
Alternative and Supplementary Methods

Once living adult worms are identified in any lymphatic vessel or lymph
node, the diagnosis of active bancroftian filariasis infection is confirmed.
In cases where only lymphangiectasia is found, a search for circulating
antigen is advised (Og4C3 test or ICT card). These tests are already available commercially. Also, a "provocative test" with diethylcarbamazine is
an alternate way to reveal the hidden adult worms in lymphatic vessels (especially in the intrascrotal vessels through the detection of small nodules
perceived by physical examination up to 7 days after treatment). This is
especially useful where vessel dilation is not enough to allow visualization
of living worms by ultrasound.

3.3.4.9
Diagnostic Efficiency

In summary, ultrasound is a very useful tool for complementing the diagnosis of bancroftian filariasis and for documenting the extension of the

lymphatic vessel damage. Its use to monitor absence of lymphangiectasia in areas where transmission has been interrupted deserves further investigation.

Acknowledgement. We thank Dr. David Addiss for reviewing the manuscript, and the NGO (Non-governmental organization) Amaury Coutinho and the World Health Organization for financial support for the bancroftian ultrasonographic studies in Brazil.

3.3.5
Liver Trematode Infection (Liver Distosomiasis)
(by Joon-Koo Han)

Distosomiasis is a group of parasitoses due to flat worms that live in contact with epithelia. Clinical classification depends on the organ infected by adults: liver, lungs, or intestines.

Liver flukes

- *Fasciola hepatica* is cosmopolitan. It is contracted when eating contaminated food (wild watercress, dandelion leaves, or lamb's lettuce, on which larvae are encysted).
- *Fasciola gigantica* or giant fluke is only found in tropical areas.
- *Dicrocoelium dendriticum* or small fluke is exceptional in humans; however, eggs are frequently found in stools.
- *Clonorchis sinensis* and *Opisthorchis viverrini* are found in the Orient.
- *Opisthorchis felineus* can be seen in Europe.

Pulmonary flukes: Mainly present in the tropics, they are extremely frequent in Far East. Freshwater crustaceans spread the infection:

- *Paragonimus westermani*
- *Paragonimus kellicoti*
- *Paragonimus africanus*

Intestinal flukes: Several species are responsible for the disease: *Fasciolopsis buski* is oriental, and can be contracted by eating water chestnuts; *Metagonimus yokogawai* is also oriental.

- *Heterophyes heterophyes* is more cosmopolitan, and can be contracted by eating raw fish.

We present as an example clonorchiasis disease.

3.3.5.1
Clonorchiasis

Epidemiology

Clonorchis sinensis infection is endemic in the Far East, especially southern China, Hong Kong, and Korea. The custom of eating slices of raw freshwater fish contributes to the high incidence of infection in these countries.

Despite a gradual decrease in prevalence over the recent decades, in 1986, it was estimated that about 15 million people were infected in the world, and a national survey in Korea in 1997 revealed that the prevalence of clonorchiasis was still 1.4%. *C. sinensis* is still the most prevalent human parasitic helminth by stool examination recently in Korea. The difficulty of eliminating clonorchiasis in the endemic area has been attributed mainly to the difficulty of detecting infected cases, although other contributory factors including re-infection after treatment have been discussed.

The rate of infection with clonorchiasis in endemic areas is greater in older patients than in younger ones. Men are more commonly infected than women. The higher percentage of clonorchiasis in men is probably related to their dietary habits. In endemic areas, there is a tradition of eating raw freshwater fish, soaked in vinegar or red-pepper mash, as an appetizer when drinking liquor at social gatherings.

C. sinensis has a life span of 10–30 years, and this creates a problem for Asian immigrants who may develop clinical symptoms several years after leaving the endemic area. Clonorchiasis in North America has been reported in recent decades, reflecting the immigration of people from endemic areas.

Pathology

The life cycle of *C. sinensis* has been well documented. The definite hosts are humans, dogs, and other mammals. The eggs, shed by the adult worm, are deposited in the biliary tree of these animals, enter the intestine, and are passed with the feces. On reaching water, the eggs are ingested by snails. Within the snail, the eggs undergo metamorphosis, after which the cercariae erupt. The free-swimming cercariae pass from the snail and penetrate the scales of freshwater fish. After a development period of several weeks, cercariae become encysted in muscle. Humans and other fish-eating animals acquire the infection by ingesting the infected fish that are raw or inadequately cooked. With digestion, the metacercariae excyst in the duodenum, migrate into the intrahepatic biliary tree via the common

Fig. 3.58. Histopathologic findings of clonorchiasis. Note the hyperplasia of biliary epithelial cells and periductal fibrosis. Note the flukes within dilated bile duct (hematoxylin and eosin, original magnification 12.5x)

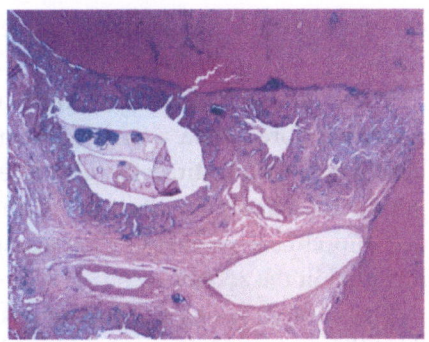

duct, and mature into adult worms (Fig. 3.58). The adult fluke inhabits the biliary tract, generally localizing within the intrahepatic bile ducts. The adult worm is a small trematode with an elliptical shape; the average worm is 10–25 mm in length. Completion of this life cycle is restricted to endemic areas, reflecting the geographic distribution of the essential snail species.

C. sinensis causes low-grade inflammatory changes in the biliary tree, severe hyperplasia of epithelial cells and metaplasia of mucopolysaccharide-producing cells in the mucosa, and progressive periductal fibrosis. The severity of these pathological changes tends to correlate with the duration of infection, the parasite burden, and the susceptibility of the host.

The cut surface of the liver reveals dilatation of the medium-sized bile ducts, with thickened walls. The histopathological findings of clonorchiasis are characterized by bile duct epithelial proliferation followed later by periductal fibrosis. Biliary hyperplasia is the distinctive lesion of early *Clonorchis* infection, but the portal tracts do not become so deranged as to lead to portal venous hypertension or biliary cirrhosis. In addition to biliary hyperplasia, the biliary epithelium frequently becomes edematous, and desquamation may be seen in areas of close proximity to the flukes. Periductal infiltrates of mononuclear cells are frequently found; however, inflammation of the bile-duct walls is generally slight in uncomplicated cases. Metaplasia of biliary epithelial cells into goblet cells occurs fairly early in infection, and these may proliferate to produce many small glandular-like structures in the mucosa, giving the bile a persistent and excessively high mucus content. Chronic and persistent infections result in a gradual increase in fibrous tissues, which may eventually engulf some of the proliferated glands, giving the appearance of cholangiofibrosis. As fibrosis proceeds, the epithelial proliferation subsides.

These histopathological changes are distinctive features of clonorchiasis. Therefore, when a variable degree of proliferation of ductal epithelium with metaplastic cells (described as adenomatous hyperplasia) and periductal fibrosis are observed in an endemic area, it is highly suggestive of clonorchiasis on histological grounds, even though the parasite is not included in the section.

The complications of clonorchiasis are the results of obstruction of the biliary system. Parasite-induced goblet cell metaplasia creates bile with a high mucin content. This bile, combined with the adult flukes and ova, serves as a nidus for bacterial superinfection and intrahepatic stone formation. The ectasia of intrahepatic bile ducts may progress to a pyogenic cholangitis, liver abscess, cholangiocarcinoma, hepatitis, and cirrhosis. Retention cysts and dilated venous radicles in the portal areas are also observed.

Many studies from endemic areas have documented the high commensurate occurrence of cholangiocarcinoma with clonorchiasis. A cause-and-effect relationship between clonorchiasis and cholangiocarcinoma is now generally accepted by most researchers, since epidemiological, experimental, and pathological data suggesting the relationship have accumulated.

Examination Technique
The patients are recommended to fast for at least four to six hours before the examination. Although it is now rare in human cases, clonorchiasis involving the gall bladder or pancreas has been reported.

Examination is in the supine position, if needed with the head elevated and the patient turned 45 degrees to the left.

The examination should always include the entire biliary system, the liver, and the pancreas. Because the sonographic diagnosis of clonorchiasis is generally made by the exclusion of obstruction in the large bile duct, the common bile duct should be completely evaluated whenever possible.

Sometimes ingestion of water (two or three cups) can improve the acoustic window for the distal common bile duct.

Color Doppler is helpful to differentiate the dilated peripheral intrahepatic ducts from accompanying portal veins.

Using a linear array transducer with high frequency (5–12 MHz) sometimes helps the depiction of ductal wall thickening and intraductal flukes.

Pathological Findings

Characteristic ultrasonographic findings of clonorchiasis are summarized as diffuse, mild, uniform dilatation of the small intrahepatic bile ducts with no dilatation, or only minimal dilatation, of larger bile ducts without a focal obstructing lesion.

The ductal wall is often thickened, and its echogenicity is increased. Occasionally, flukes or aggregates of ova can be shown as non-shadowing echogenic foci or cast within the bile duct (Figs. 3.59a–d and 3.60a–c).

These findings are considered a pathognomonic finding of clonorchiasis.

Differential Diagnosis

Differential diagnosis of clonorchiasis includes cancer along the bile ducts, choledocholithiasis with recurrent pyogenic cholangitis, sclerosing cholangitis, Caroli disease, and *Fasciola hepatica* infection.

Pitfalls

At present, clonorchiasis is commonly diagnosed incidentally during radiological screening (especially, ultrasonography) of the abdomen for other purposes, since symptoms of clonorchiasis are vague and nonspecific in most cases. The biliary dilatation observed in ultrasonography should not be misinterpreted as being caused by a focal obstructive lesion in the biliary tree, because this misinterpretation may mislead to unnecessary diagnostic tests or invasive procedures. Once diagnosed, clonorchiasis is treated very effectively with praziquantel, with few side-effects.

Efforts should be taken to find an occult cholangiocarcinoma during the examination.

Alternative and Supplementary Methods

Clonorchiasis should be suspected in a patient who develops manifestations of hepatic or biliary disease and who has a history of ingesting raw freshwater fish in an endemic area. The diagnosis of liver fluke infestation is usually established by microscopic examination of stools for ova and/or adult parasites. A formalin-ether sedimentation technique is known to be more reliable than the direct-smear method for detecting eggs in feces.

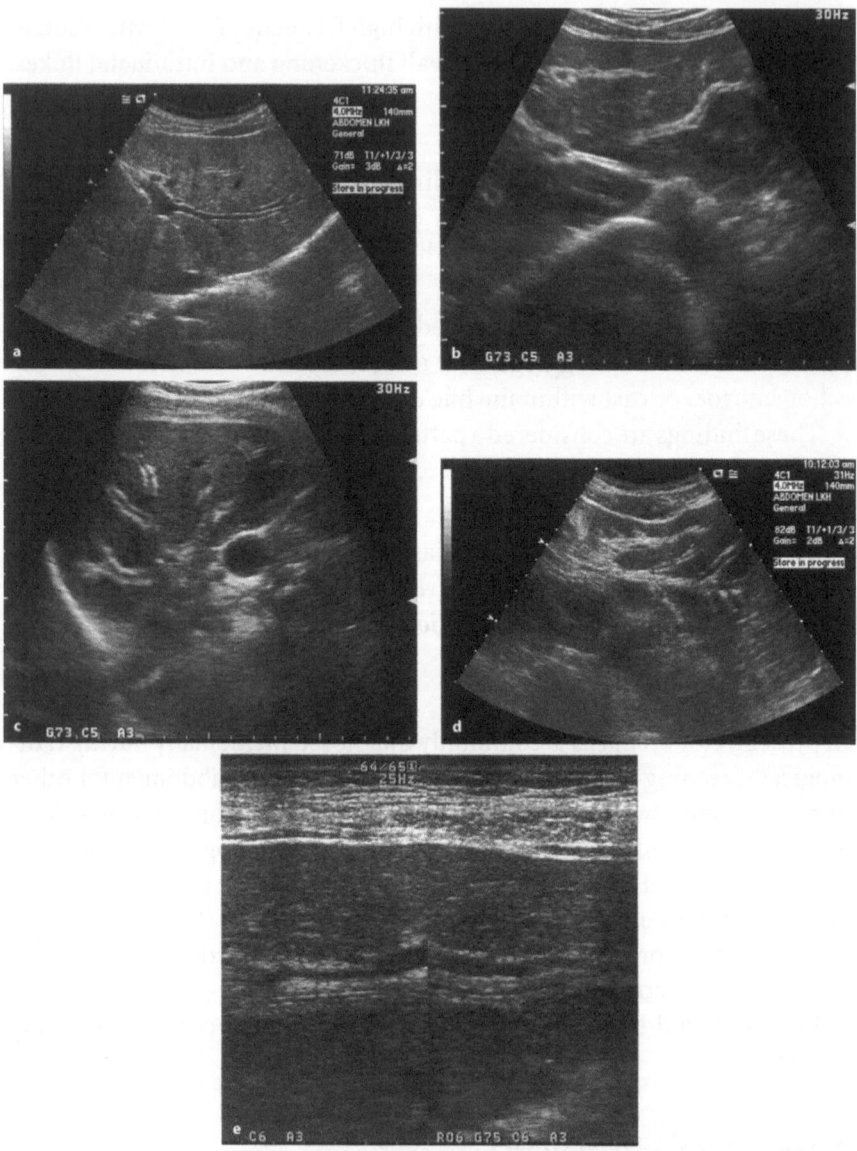

Fig. 3.59a–e. Ultrasonographic findings of clonorchiasis. Note the diffuse, mild, uniform dilatation of the small intrahepatic bile ducts with no dilatation, or only minimal dilatation, of larger bile ducts. The ductal wall is thickened, and its echogenicity is increased. Using linear transducer with high frequency helps the depiction of ductal wall thickening (e). Each figure is from a different patient

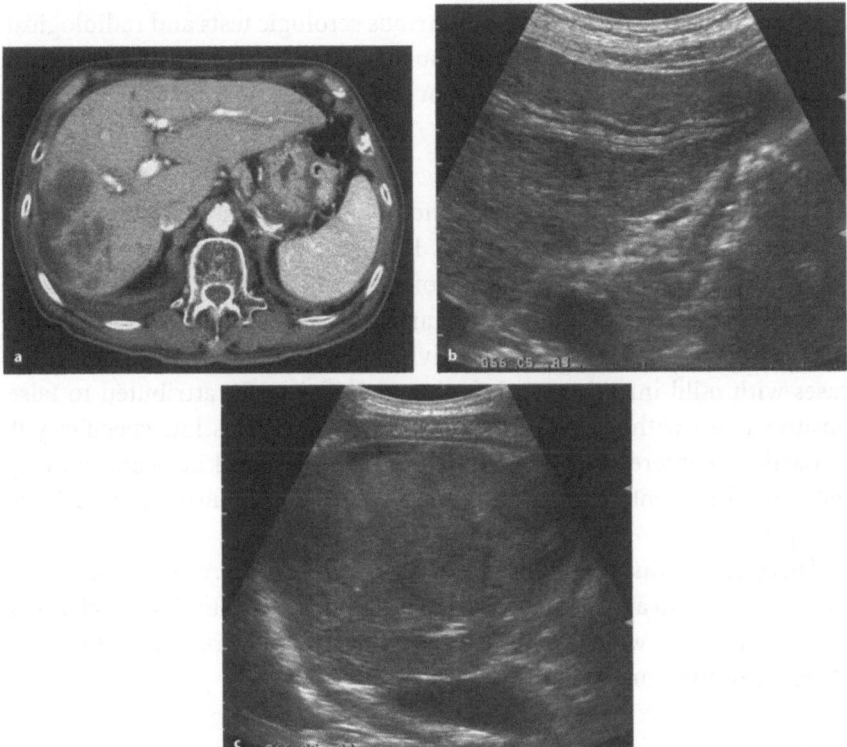

Fig. 3.60a–c. A patient with clonorchiasis-associated cholangiocarcinoma. (a) Transverse contrast-enhanced CT shows diffuse, mild, uniform dilatation of the small intrahepatic bile ducts with no dilatation, or only minimal dilatation, of larger bile ducts. (b) Transverse ultrasonography at epigastrium shows mild dilatation of the small intrahepatic bile duct at segment III. The ductal wall is thickened, and its echogenicity is increased. This finding was observed in diffuse distribution in the entire liver. (c) Right intercostals scan shows mass in the right liver

Although the diagnosis of clonorchiasis is easily made by the stool examination, mass screening with fecal examination can be more difficult, because of poor voluntary cooperation. A number of serologic techniques have been developed to aid in the diagnosis of clonorchiasis. However, unfortunately, the serologic methods currently available exhibit considerable cross-reactivity. Accordingly, they are not widely accepted as screening techniques.

Computed tomography, as well as ultrasonography, is widely accepted as an accurate and feasible diagnostic method for clonorchiasis.

Although helpful, none of these various serologic tests and radiological examinations has been reported to surpass fecal examination, because of their limited sensitivity, specificity, or applicability.

Diagnostic Efficiency
Aforementioned ultrasonographic findings are regarded as pathognomonic for clonorchiasis in endemic areas. However, more recent studies have shown the low diagnostic accuracy of ultrasonography for clonorchiasis. According to a study in an endemic area, the sensitivity was 52% and the specificity was 51%; the low sensitivity was attributed to false negative cases with mild infection, and the low specificity was attributed to false positive cases with residual pathology after cure. This low specificity is of particular interest, since the number of cases cured has continuously increased in recent decades, because of nationwide control and ecologic changes.

Therefore, ultrasonography is less useful for the differentiation of cured clonorchiasis and active infection, since it reflects the pathological changes in the bile ducts, which may persist for years after cure, rather than the presence of the worm itself.

3.3.6
Schistosomiasis
(by Maria C. Chammas, Ilka R.S. de Oliveira, Giovanni G. Cerri)

Schistosomiasis is a parasitic disease of slow progression caused by trematodes of the genus Schistosoma, first described in the mid-19th century by the German pathologist Theodor Bilharz. It is an important public health problem in certain regions of the world, including South America, the Caribbean, Africa, and the Middle East. It is estimated that approximately 250 million individuals are infected in 76 countries, and that 500 to 600 million people are exposed to the infection.

The most prevalent species of the Schistosoma are: *Schistosoma mansoni*, *Schistosoma japonicum*, and *Schistosoma haematobium*, with the two first species associated with the hepatosplenic form of the illness and the latter species with the genitourinary form.

The World Health Organization (WHO) recently proposed a standardization of the use of diagnostic ultrasound in schistosomiasis indicated for field studies. For epidemiological purposes, it is very important that ultrasound examinations be carried out and recorded in a standardized way, to ensure that results obtained in different places at different times can be compared. This standardization has been used in several countries in endemic areas.

The most important clinical signs are related to portal hypertension in *S. mansoni* and *S. japonicum* and to kidney function impairment in *S. haematobium*.

3.3.6.1
Schistosoma mansoni

The hepatosplenic form of Manson's schistosomiasis affects the liver, spleen, gall bladder, the portal system, and its tributaries.

The advanced hepatosplenic form is identified 5–10 years after the initial infection, being associated with the development of periportal fibrosis and portal hypertension. In the absence of other hepatic diseases, such as hepatitis caused by the B and C virus, the inflammatory process resulting from schistosomiasis usually does not affect the hepatic cellular parenchyma, so that no significant alterations in the hepatic function can be observed. However, portal hypertension leads to repeated bouts of hematemesis secondary to esophageal and gastric varices, a dreadful complication and a cause of morbidity.

Other clinical manifestations caused by intestinal schistosome infection are glomerulonephritis, functional alterations of the exocrine pancreas, and pulmonary hypertension.

Due to the hemorrhages in the upper digestive tract, repetitive blood transfusions are carried out. Consequently, the association with viral cirrhosis (for virus B or C) is not uncommon, so that the overlapping of the findings of viral cirrhosis or even hepatocarcinoma with those of schistosomiasis should be considered.

Pathophysiology
After penetrating the skin, the parasites, in the form of cercariae, are carried to the lung, and they reach the liver through the systemic circulation, where they mature and males and females pair off. Subsequently, they migrate against the blood flow to the mesenteric veins and to the bowel submucosa, where the egg-laying takes place.

The evolution of the illness in the liver is carried out through the parasite's egg embolization from the bowel submucosa to the venous portal

Fig. 3.61. Macroscopic examination of the liver, showing intense fibrous periportal thickening

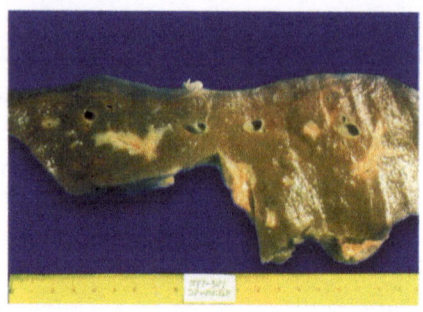

circulation. The inflammatory reaction to the presence of the eggs (and sometimes to the dead parasite as well) leads to the formation of chronic epithelial granulomas and to Symmer's periportal fibrosis. With the disease evolution, the periportal fibrosis progresses and establishes a venous obstruction, contributing to the state of presinusoidal portal hypertension. Macroscopically, the liver presents an increase of the left lobe, atrophy of the right lobe, blunt borders, and fibrous thickening of the portal spaces of up to 3 cm. The fibrous periportal thickening is more intense in the hepatic hilum, extending in varying degrees to the portal intrahepatic spaces and to the perivesicular region.

Additionally, the spleen may be enlarged to over 650 g in 50% of the patients, presenting sinusoidal dilatation, hemorrhages, and later formation of siderotic nodules (Gamna-Gandi bodies) (Fig. 3.63).

Diagnostic Imaging

The morphologic and biometric aspects of the hepatosplenic form of schistosomiasis can be studied by several diagnostic imaging methods, such as Doppler ultrasonography (US-Doppler), scintigraphy, computerized tomography (CT scanning), splenoportography, and magnetic resonance imaging (MRI). The US-Doppler evaluation presents the advantages of noninvasiveness and of being accessible to the majority of the patients, becoming an important step in the practice of modern diagnostic medicine. Thus, this method has been also applied in a series of epidemiological studies, in those regions of high prevalence. The morphologic and hemodynamic parameters obtained by this method make both the diagnosis of portal hypertension and its vascular complications possible.

US-Doppler Aspects

The anatomical-pathological aspects previously described can be recognized by means of US-Doppler study, preceding, sometimes, the beginning of the clinical manifestations of the illness. It is important to point out that US-Doppler is useful not only for the diagnosis but for the follow-up of the clinical treatment. In the initial phases of hepatosplenic schistosomiasis, discrete and nonspecific alterations are observed, such as hepatomegaly without periportal thickening, making the characterization of the disease difficult.

The volumetric alterations of the liver, remarkably the increase of the left hepatic lobe and the reduction of the right hepatic lobe, are observed in the hepatosplenic schistosomiasis (Fig. 3.62). These alterations can easily be characterized by B-mode ultrasonography, as can the splenomegaly with the Gamna-Gandi bodies. The siderotic nodules are evidenced as dispersed hyperechogenic points in the splenic parenchyma. However, due to their dimensions (3–15 mm), they are only observed in up to 7% of the patients (Fig. 3.63).

The fibrous periportal thickening is one of the morphologic features that allows the recognition of the illness, being characterized on ultrasonography as a band of periportal hyperechogenicity in about 73–100% of the cases. This thickening mainly affects the portal vein at the hepatic hilum, and also extends to the intrahepatic portal branches and the perivesicular region (Figs. 3.64, 3.65). However, in the initial phase of the illness, the periportal fibrosis is difficult to characterize by ultrasound. Periportal fibrosis causes an increase in venous pressure in the splanchnic territory, constituting the presinusoidal portal hypertension. As a consequence, an

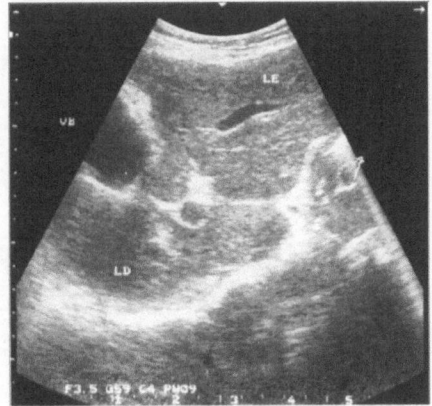

Fig. 3.62. Volumetric alterations of the liver, remarkable increase of the left hepatic lobe, and reduction of the right hepatic lobe

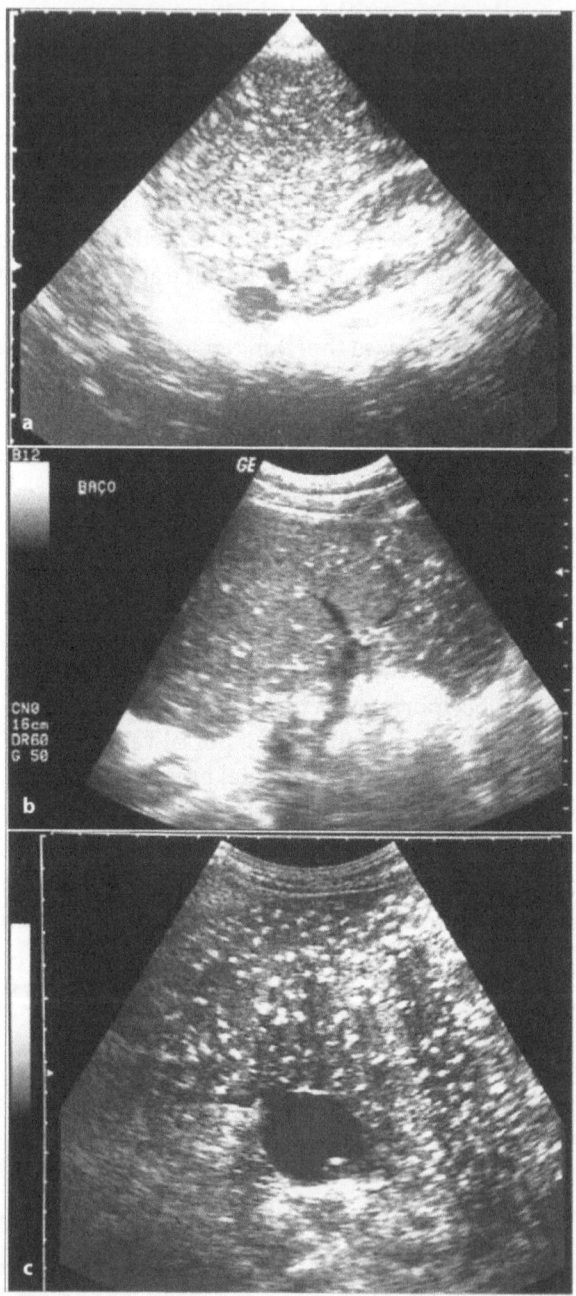

Fig. 3.63a–c. Splenomegaly with Gamna-Gandi bodies (hyperechogenic points in the splenic parenchyma)

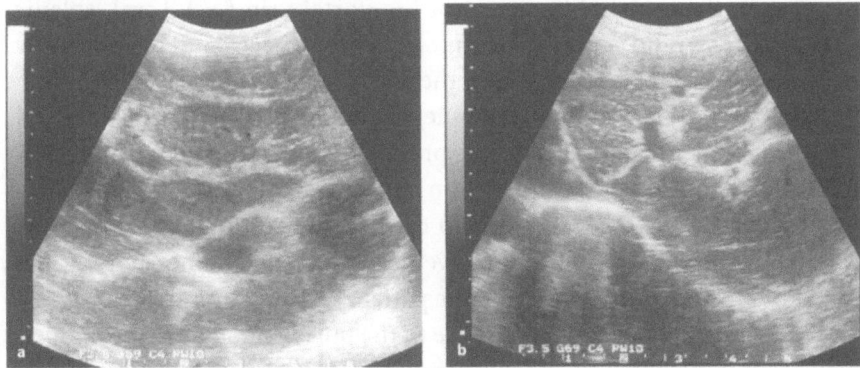

Fig. 3.64a,b. Fibrous periportal thickening at the hepatic hilum and intrahepatic portal branches

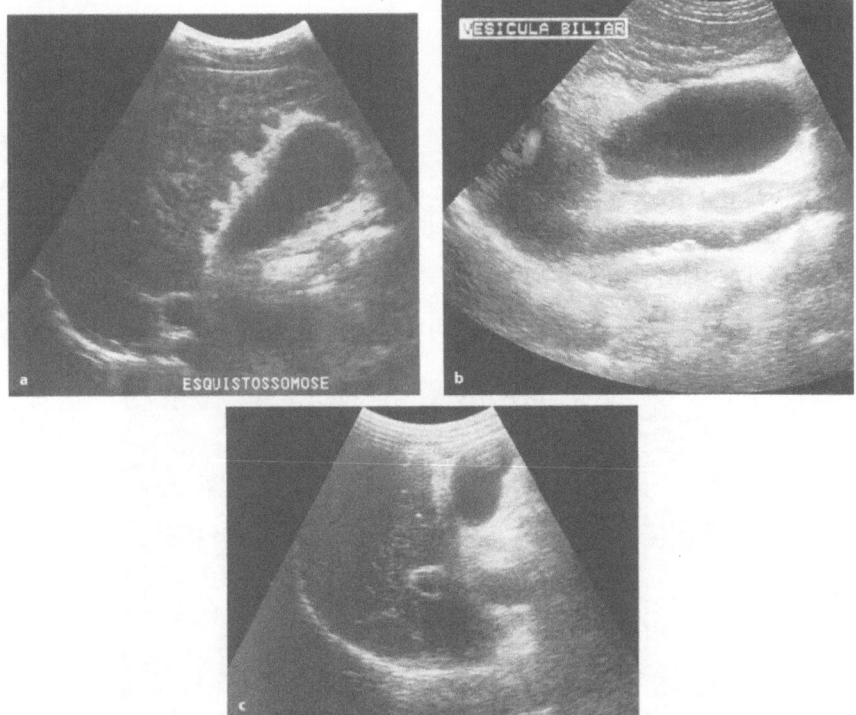

Fig. 3.65a–c. Fibrous periportal thickening at the hepatic hilum and perivesicular region

increase in the caliber (diameter) of the portal vein (> 1.2 cm), splenic
vein (> 0.9 cm), and superior mesenteric vein (> 0.9 cm) can be frequently
observed in 73%, 68%, and 42% of the cases, respectively (Fig. 3.66).

An analysis by color duplex-Doppler generally discloses the hepatopetal
flow direction in the portal vein, preserved spectral tracing morphology, and blood flow velocity within the normal standards. Some flow
oscillations can be observed, due to cardiac and respiratory movements
(Fig. 3.67). Thrombosis of the portal vein is a rather uncommon finding, being found in approximately 6% of the patients. However, with the progressive increase of the hepatic resistance to the portal blood flow, thrombosis
may occur in the main portal stem and/or in its branches, filling its lumen
with echogenic material, partially or completely obstructing the vessel.
Even though the Doppler color mapping does not display the blood flow

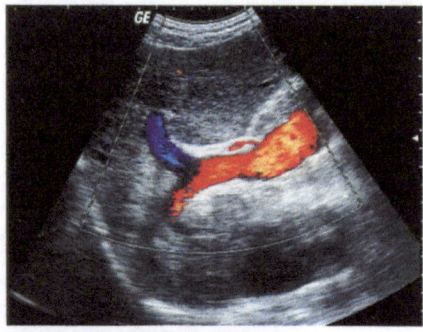

Fig. 3.66. Portal hypertension causes increase in the diameter of portal vein
(1.4 cm)

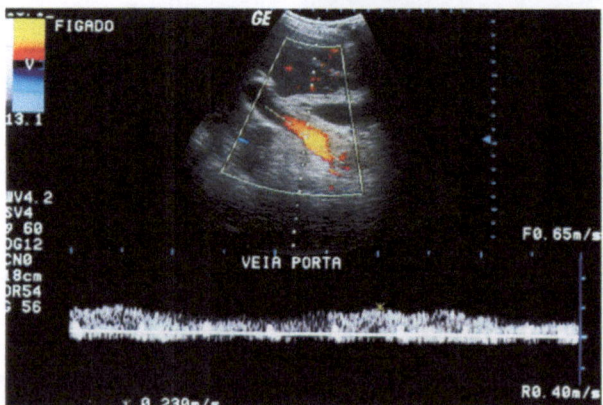

Fig. 3.67. Color duplex-Doppler scan showing hepatopetal flow direction in the portal
vein, preserved spectral tracing morphology, and blood flow velocity (23 cm/sec)

in the presence of complete thrombosis, in the partial thrombosis events, flow becomes evident in the vein's peripheral region (Figs. 3.68–3.70).

In the cases of chronic thrombosis, cavernous transformation of the portal vein may occur, being represented by the identification of collateral circulation in this anatomic region (see Fig. 3.72). US-Doppler demonstrates an elongated echogenic structure, pervaded by serpiginous images with low-velocity monophasic flow, without the resulting fluctuating alterations of the cardiac cycle.

The portal thrombosis can also occur as a complication of esophageal varices sclerotherapy, bypass surgeries (mesenteric-cava, porto-caval, dis-

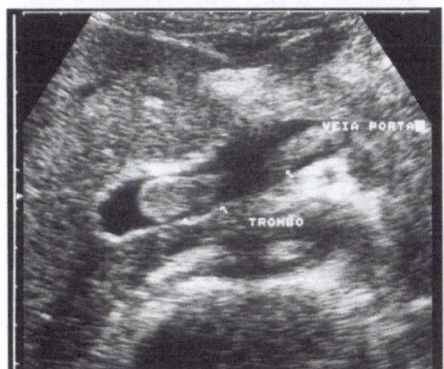

Fig. 3.68. Partially portal thrombosis, with echogenic material inside the portal vein

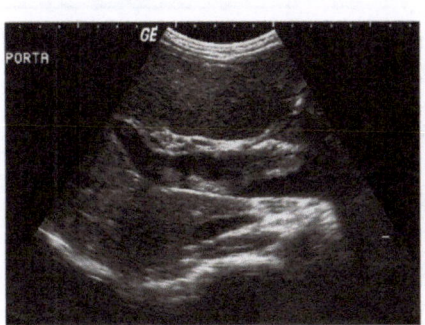
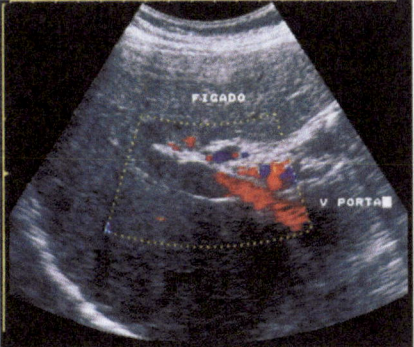

Fig. 3.69. Complete portal thrombosis, with hypoechogenic material inside the portal vein (recent thrombosis)

Fig. 3.70. Power Doppler scan showing complete portal thrombosis (chronic) and identifying collateral circulation in this anatomic region, pervaded by serpiginous images (cavernous transformation)

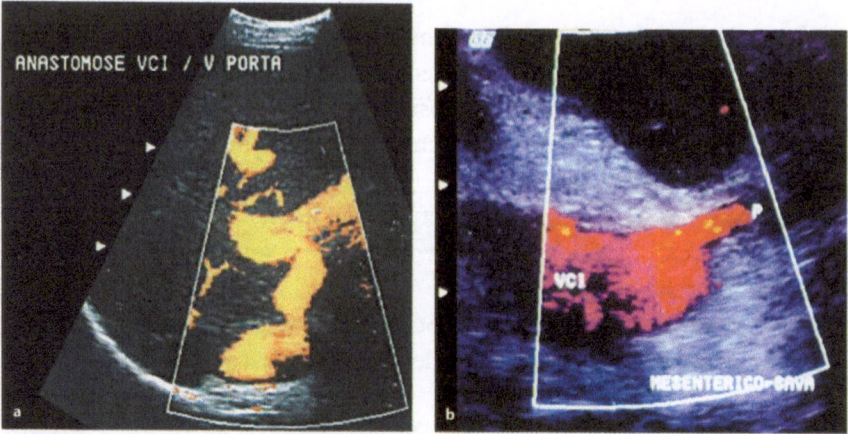

Fig. 3.71a,b. Spontaneous splenorenal anastomosis, demonstrated by color Doppler scan

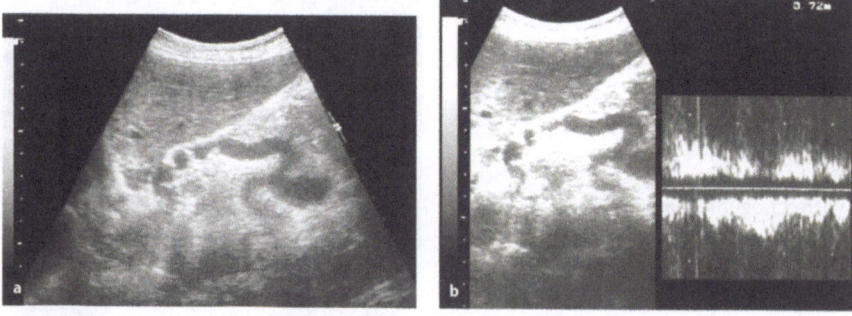

Fig. 3.72a,b. Venous collateral circulation (dilated left gastric vein). B-scan and Doppler

tal splenorenal) (Fig. 3.71), or disconnecting surgeries (azygo-portal and splenectomy).

US-Doppler studies of the splenic vein and superior mesenteric vein demonstrate an increase in their caliber/diameter in several degrees, with hepatopetal flow direction, spectral tracing, and maximum velocities within the normality standards. However, in the presence of splenorenal anastomosis, the splenic vein (and eventually the portal vein) can present flow in the reverse direction (hepatofugal flow) (Fig. 3.32). Another common finding is the presence of venous collateral circulation, evidenced in 36–78% of the patients. These vessels can be identified in hepatic hilum, at the small gastric curve (left or coronary gastric vein) (Fig. 3.72), in the fundus of the stomach (short gastric veins) (Fig. 3.73), along the round ligament (paraumbilical vein) (Fig. 3.74), around the gall bladder (cystic

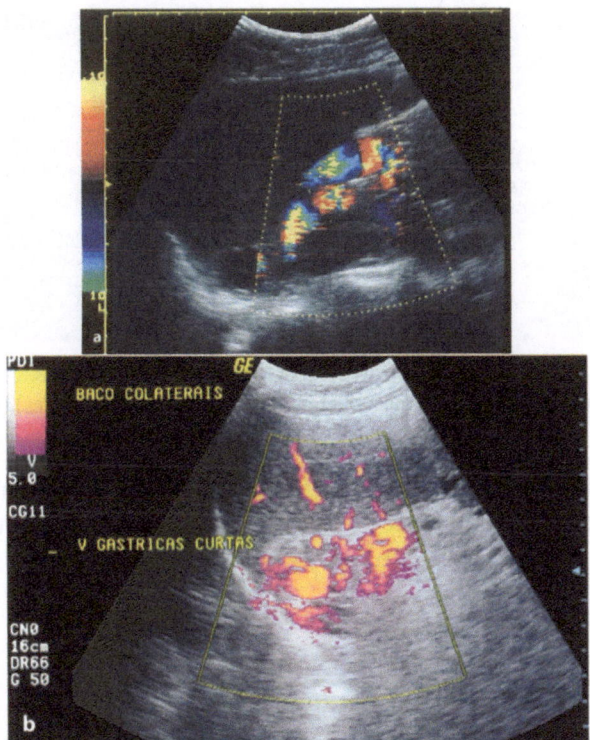

Fig. 3.73a,b. Color Doppler scan (**a**) and power Doppler (**b**) showing the venous collateral circulation (short gastric veins)

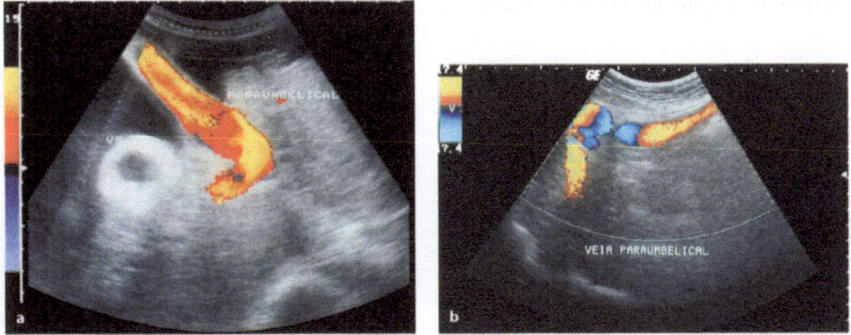

Fig. 3.74a,b. Color Doppler scan showing the venous collateral circulation with hepatofugal flow in the paraumbilical vein

varices) (Fig. 3.75), and in other retroperitoneal sites (for example, spontaneous splenorenal anastomosis) (Fig. 3.71). The collateral circulation generally presents hepatofugal flow. Finally, the hepatic veins can display

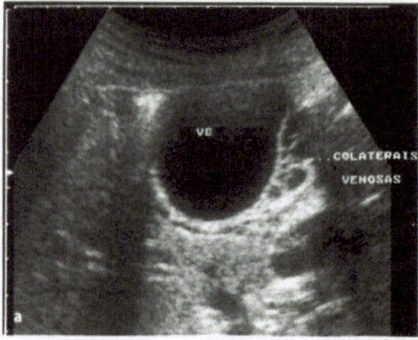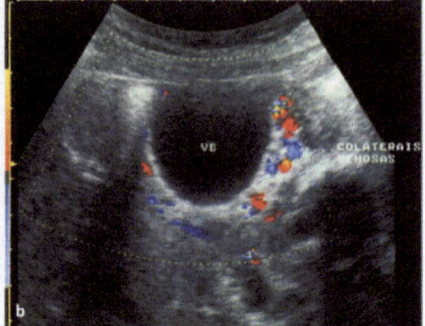

Fig. 3.75a,b. Perivesicular fibrosis, represented by hyperechogenic tissue (a) and Color Doppler scan showing the venous collateral circulation (cystic varices) (b)

alterations in the spectral tracing as a result of the reduction of the hepatic parenchyma compliance due to the fibrosis, presenting a two-phase or single-phase flow ("portalized").

3.3.6.2
Schistosoma japonicum

Many lesions due to *S. japonicum* are similar to those of *S. mansoni*.

There are particular fibrous changes in the liver parenchyma different from those of *S. mansoni*, giving the architecture a more prominent network of fibrosis (fish scales) (Fig. 3.76).

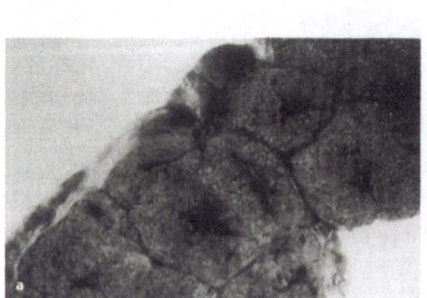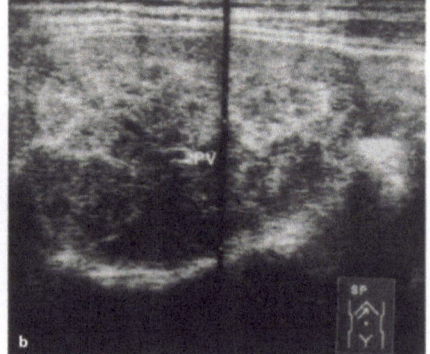

Fig. 3.76a,b. *S. japonicum.* **a** Fibrosis, typical aspect of fish scales. **b** Periportal fibrosis suggesting the fish scales aspect

3.3.6.3
Schistosoma haematobium

The alterations in this genito-urinary form are found mainly in the kidneys, the ureters, and the bladder. The severity and frequency of the lesions are related to the intensity of the infection.

Obstructive uropathy that varies from mild to severe, with reduction of the thickness of the renal parenchyma, is a common sign. Bands of fibrosis (hyperechoic band) are an additional finding in the kidneys. The stage of hydronephrosis indicates the severity of the disease.

Dilatation of the ureter could be very important; it is easily identified with ultrasound (Fig. 3.77).

The most important findings, in the bladder, are as follows: thickening and irregularity of the wall with development of pseudopolyps and masses and calcifications (Fig. 3.78).

Liver abnormalities, similar to those related in *S. mansoni*, may also be observed.

Ultrasound is very important in the follow-up of portal hypertension, demonstrating the course of the disease or reduction of periportal fibrosis after treatment. Doppler could be used to monitor changes in portal flow after treatment. In urinary schistosomiasis, the affected bladder and kidneys could be evaluated.

The differential diagnosis includes a chronic liver disease with portal hypertension for *S. mansoni* and *S. japonicum* and inflammatory (particularly tuberculosis), obstructive and tumoral lesions for *S. haematobium*. When the bowel lesion is identified, the differential diagnosis is with granulomatous or ulcerative colitis and tumoral polyps. In the lung, other causes of interstitial pattern and pulmonary hypertension should be considered.

Usually, the diagnostic presentation of schistosomiasis is very characteristic and specific.

Ultrasound is definitively adopted as an epidemiologic tool in schistosomiasis.

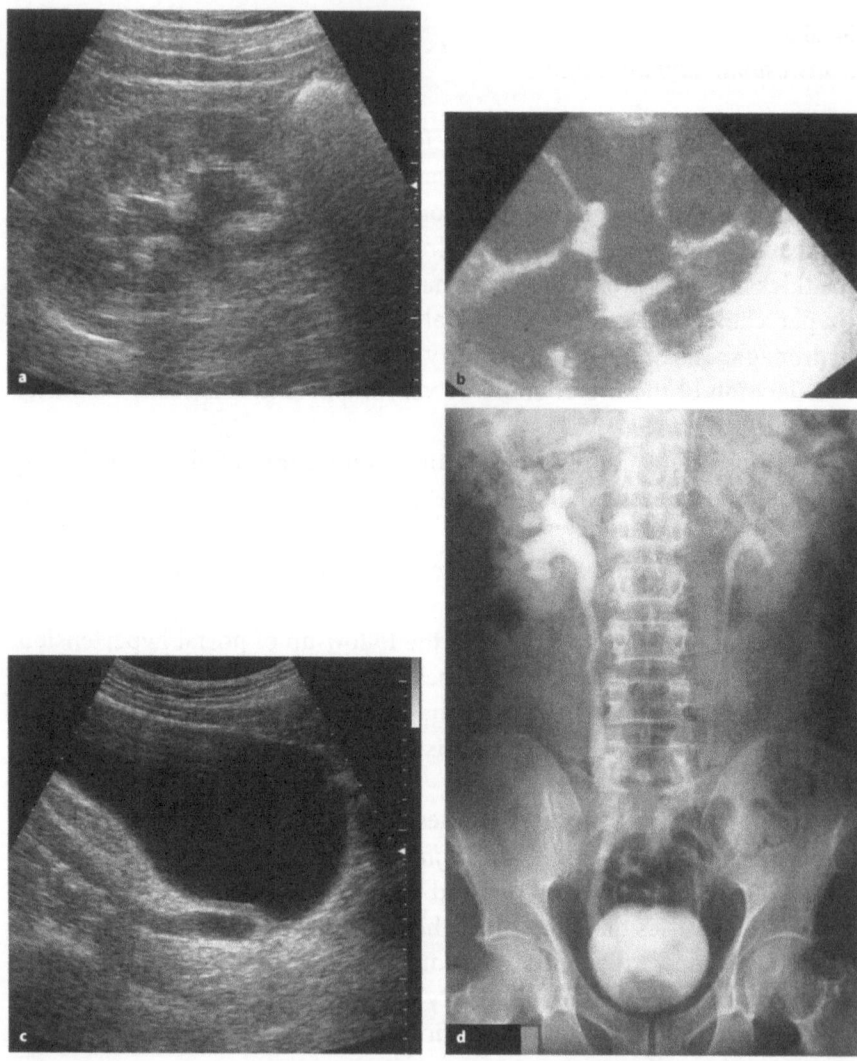

Fig. 3.77a–d. *S. haematobium.* **a** Discrete dilatation of the renal cavities. **b** Important hydronephrosis. **c** Dilated pelvis ureter. **d** IVP same patient as in Fig. 3.24c

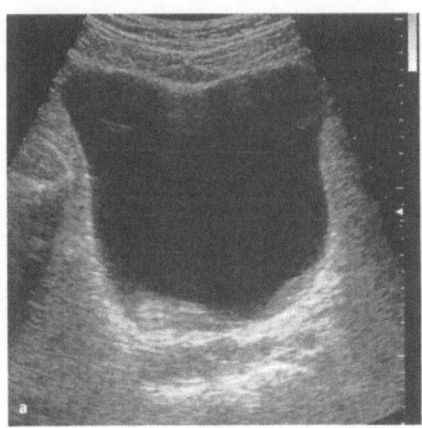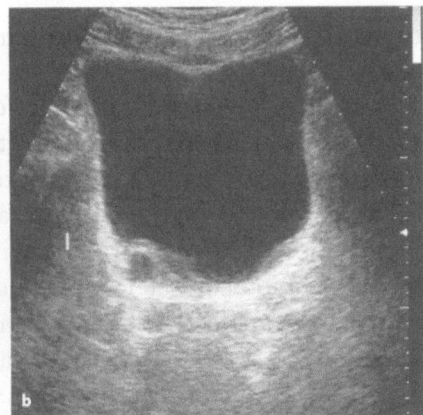

Fig. 3.78a,b. *S. haematobium*. a Localized thickening of the bladder wall, pseudo masse aspect. b Pseudo polyp aspect. c Bladder wall calcification

3.3.7
Echinococcosis

3.3.7.1
Hydatid Disease
(by Ferid Ben Chehida, Heykel Ben Romdhane, Azza Hammou, Hassen A. Gharbi)

Hydatid disease is caused by *Echinococcus granulosus*; this cestodiasis of cosmopolitan distribution occurs predominantly in areas of intensive sheep or cattle farming.

Humans are an accidental host in the animal parasitosis which involves two hosts: a definitive, carnivorous host (usually a dog) and an intermediate herbivorous animal (sheep, cattle, camel). The adult tapeworm lives in the jejunum of the dog; the eggs it releases are passed in the excreta; when ingested by an intermediate host, they reach the stomach, and the embryos released penetrate the intestinal wall and reach the liver through the portal system. The larvae are carried to the lungs, and get into the general circulation; no part of the organism is protected from infestation. The larvae rapidly become surrounded by an inflammatory granuloma and transform into a multinuclear protoplasmic mass that develops over a week into a vesicle or hydatid. Over a period of 16 to 20 weeks, the cyst doubles in size as it becomes filled with fluid. This period of progressive development leads to the production of thousands of scolices; at the same time, an intense tissue reaction around the vesicle results in the formation of a tough wall called the pericyst.

If the intermediate herbivorous host dies and the cyst-containing flesh is eaten by a dog, each scolex grows to an adult worm in the dog jejunum. Like intermediate hosts, humans become infected more often during close contact with dogs (hands licked by an infected animal, or hands brought into contact with the mouth after having touched an infected dog) than after ingestion of food or water contaminated by the excreta of infected dogs.

The geographic distribution of hydatid disease is wide and includes South America, Australia, New Zealand, East and especially North Africa, and the Mediterranean area. Certain occupations are particularly exposed to the risk of contracting hydatidosis: these are shepherds and sheep farmers, veterinarians and laboratory personnel, butchers and meat packers.

All the organs may be affected, but, in adult age, the liver (60%) and the lungs (20%) are the sites of predilection. The majority of the cases, except for the liver, are primary, following vascular dissemination. There is no sex predilection. Infestation may occur at any age, generally from 2 years onwards. Most cases are seen in young adults.

The clinical manifestations of abdominal hydatidosis are variable, and depend on the location and the stage of development of the parasite: abdominal mass, abdominal pain, hepatomegaly (with or without jaundice), and ascites. Sometimes its discovery is fortuitous, during systematic exploration for a lung location or during an epidemiologic study in an endemic area.

Ultrasound Findings

Several classifications have been proposed to present ultrasound findings, based on the sonographic analysis of the morphology and structure of

Table 3.1. WHO proposed classification of cystic echinococcosis: Six types

WHO	CL	CE 1	CE 2	CE 3	CE 4	CE 5
Gharbi	+ / – I	I	III	IV	IV	V
Caremani	I-a	I-a,b	II-a,b	III-a,b, IV	V-a,b	VI-a,b
Perdomoo	I	I	II	III	IV-a	V, VI

CL, cystic lesion, nonspecific CE, cystic echinococcosis
I, II: active
III: transitional
IV, V: inactive

the hydatid cyst corresponding to its various developmental stages. The most common worldwide used is the Gharbi classification, with five types of sonographic patterns, described in 1981, which is simple and can be adopted for the description of US, CT and MR images. For the future, the WHO informal working group on cystic Echinococcosis is trying to unify the most important proposed classifications (Table 3.1).

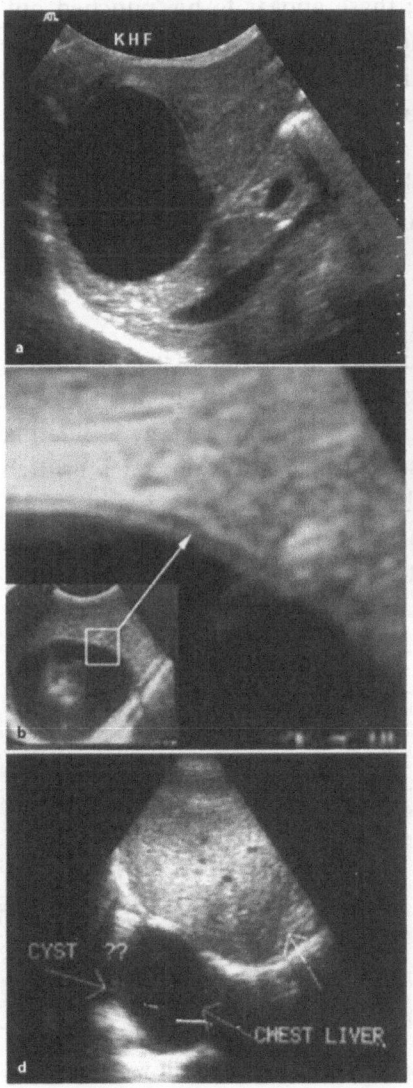

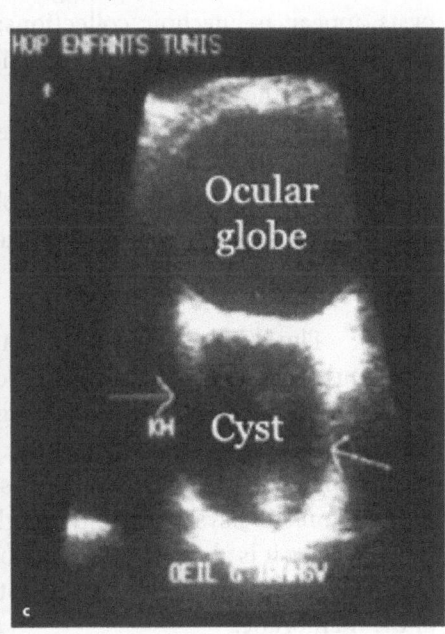

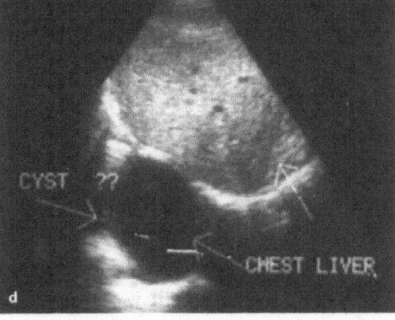

Fig. 3.79a–d. a Liver hydatid cyst type I: pure fluid collection. **b** Liver hydatid cyst type I: See the localized thickening of the cyst wall very suggestive of HC. **c** Orbit US: retro-ocular hydatid cyst. **d** Chest hydatid cyst

Gharbi Classification

Type I: Pure Fluid Collection (Fig. 3.79).

This type appears as an anechoic space with marked enhancement of back-wall echoes. The fluid collection is rounded with well-defined borders; its walls often vary in thickness. This localized thickening should be sought systematically, and is a very suggestive sign of a hydatid cyst. Only small cysts appear as anechoic collections; these appear to be 'punched out' and do not show proper walls on echography. Some cysts situated at the periphery of the liver, or the spleen, in contact with the abdominal wall or the diaphragm, are no longer rounded but oval-shaped and seem to follow the parietal contours. The size of the cysts varies greatly, from 1 to 20 cm in diameter. The pure fluid collection is the most notable aspect. The liquid is clear, and corresponds to cysts that are new, monovesicular, and noncomplicated.

Type II: Fluid Collection with a Split Wall (Fig. 3.80)

The fluid collection retains its well-defined contour but it is often less rounded, and appears to be 'sagging' in places. The split wall may be localized in an area just outside the cyst, or it may become a 'floating membrane' loose inside the cyst. This splitting of the wall, which is often discreet, must be systematically sought in any intrahepatic liquid collection, because it is almost pathognomonic for a hydatid cyst. The split wall may result from a lowering of intracystic pressure, causing the detachment of the membrane.

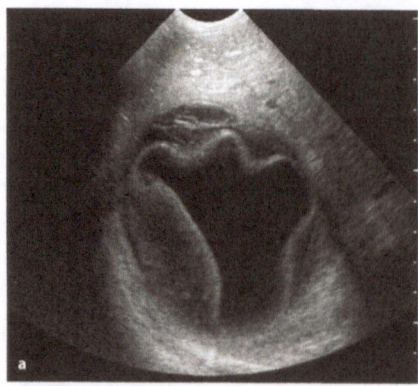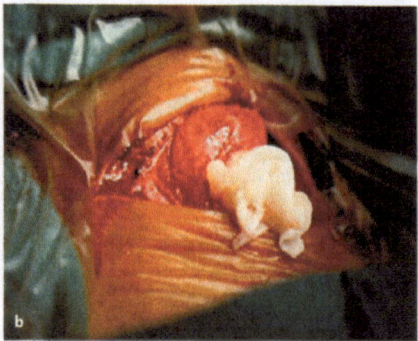

Fig. 3.80a,b. a Liver hydatid cyst type II: fluid collection with a split wall.**b** Thyroid hydatid cyst; see the membrane

Type III: Fluid Collection with Septa (Fig. 3.81)
The fluid collection retains its well-defined contour, but it is divided by
septa which are more or less thick and complete, forming oval-shaped
or rounded structures. The enhancement of back-wall echoes is usually
evident. The most typical cases show a 'honeycomb' image. The echoes
within the cysts show images of simple or multiple secondary vesicles.
When characteristic, the sonographic appearance of the secondary vesicles allows diagnosis of hydatid cysts. However, this diagnosis is sometimes
difficult to affirm. Intracystic septation may take another aspect: it may
delineate masses of various shapes that are not rounded, but show undu-
lated contours. This appearance is due to the folding of the detached cystic
membrane.

Type IV: Heterogeneous Echo Patterns (Fig. 3.82).
This type of cyst appears as a roughly rounded mass, with irregular contours and echo pattern. We have found three general pattern types:
    IV-1: hypoechoic appearance with a few irregular echoes, always due to
infected multilocular cysts
    IV-2: hyperechoic solid pattern without back-wall shadow, and
    IV-3: intermediate pattern including both hypoechoic structures and
hyperechoic structures in approximately equal quantity, the latter being
clustered in nodular patterns.
    Since it is difficult to make a diagnosis from these structures, it is
necessary to look for other diagnostic signs of hydatid cysts, such as
a membrane seen as a linear ribbon or band pattern, variable appearance
of echographic images from one section to another in the same area,
hyperechoic contour with possible areas of acoustic shadow, presence of
small fluid collections from intra or extracystic secondary vesicles, or the
presence of another cyst at a different stage of development, in the liver or
in another organ.

Type V: Reflecting Thick Walls (Fig. 3.83)
This type appears as a formation with a very hyperechoic contour, and
with a cone-shaped shadow which is usually outlined to some degree.
When this formation is small, we can visualize the whole contour. When it
is bigger, only its immediate front wall is visualized: this appears as a thick
arch-shaped image with a posterior concavity.

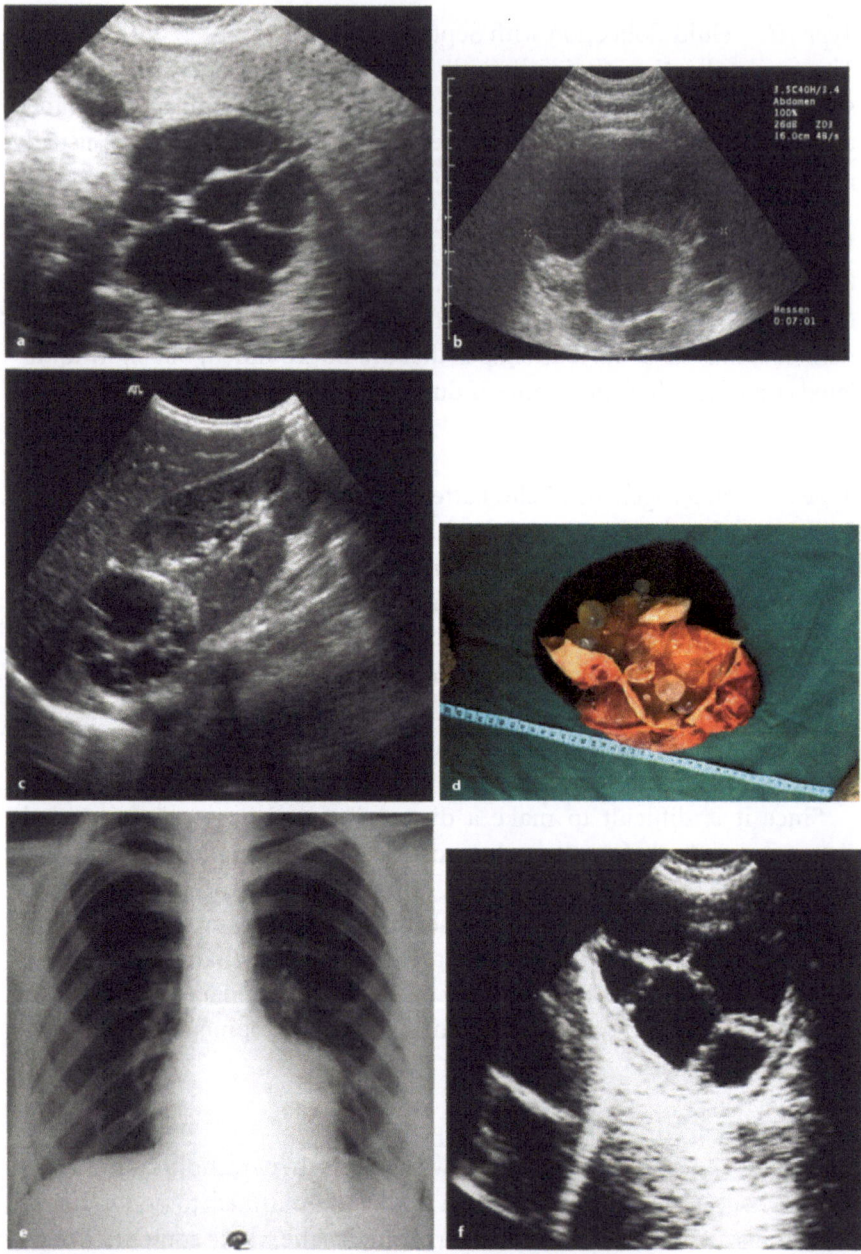

Fig. 3.81a–f. a Liver hydatid cyst type III: Fluid collection with septa. **b** Renal hydatid cyst type III. **c** Renal hydatid cyst, see daughter vesicles (same patient as in **b**). **d** Chest X-ray: Left ventricle heart hydatid cyst. **e** Heart US: hydatid cyst Type III (same patient as in **d**). **f** Macroscopic post mortem study (same patient as in **e**)

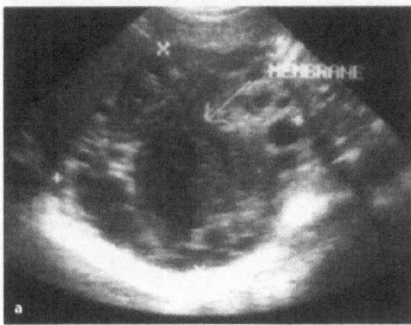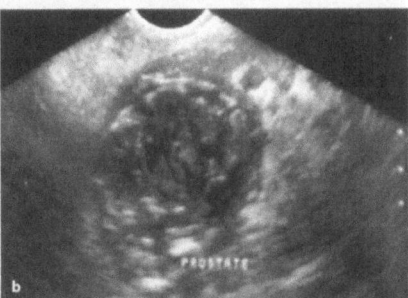

Fig. 3.82. a Liver hydatid cyst type IV: heterogeneous echo patterns.**b** Prostate hydatid cyst, a very rare localization

Fig. 3.83. Liver hydatid cyst type V: reflecting thick wall

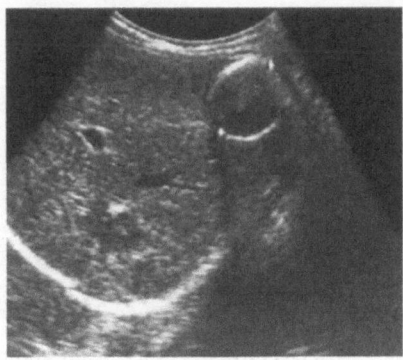

Complicated Hydatid Cyst, Other Patterns

The natural evolution of a hydatid cyst is difficult to predict. Sometimes it may develop into a calcified mass or produce compression of adjacent organs cavities and vessels, e.g., inferior vena cava, portal and hepatic veins, biliary tract, urinary tract. The cyst may rupture or become infected. In the liver, for instance, the most frequent complication is cyst rupture into the biliary ducts, through the diaphragm, or into the peritoneum. In these cases, ultrasound may show a dilated biliary tract with fragments of membranes in the gall bladder or in the common biliary duct, Budd Chiari syndrome with compression of the hepatic veins by hydatid cyst (Fig. 3.84), multiple peritoneal cyst, ascites, and, in some cases, diaphragmatic breach with a communicant supradiaphragmatic space (Fig. 3.85)

In all these cases, we can see other less frequent patterns, for example very hyperechoic masses corresponding to the shell cyst, which is usually

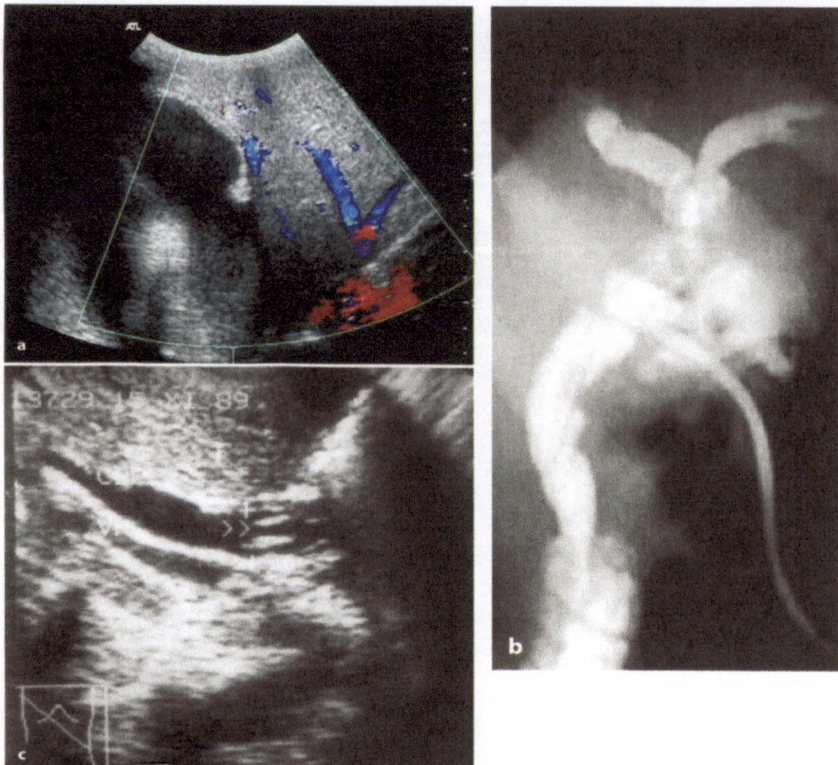

Fig. 3.84. a Liver hydatid cyst causing compression of the hepatic veins (color Doppler). **b** Hydatid cyst ruptured into the biliary ducts. Note the hydatid membranes. **c** Hydatid cyst ruptured into the biliary ducts. Note the hydatid membrane inside the main biliary duct. (courtesy of Dr. Badea, Romania)

calcified to some degree. In liquid collection, some declivitous echoes may appear and represent hydatid sand (Fig. 3.86).

Other Modalities

In endemic areas, ultrasound plays the main role, in general, among the imaging modalities. However, conventional X-ray is a very important tool for the chest and bone location; but, for the intracranial and spine location, CT and MRI, when available, are necessary. These new modalities, with multislice technique and sophisticated reconstructions, permit a better overall view of the size, location, and number of cysts within the affected organs, and vascular relationships.

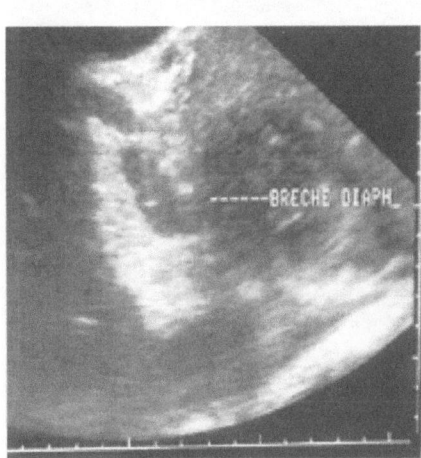 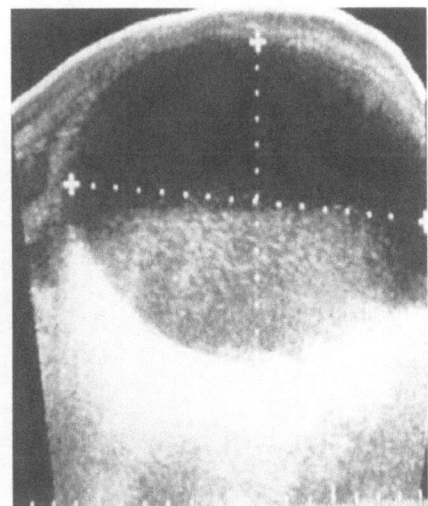

Fig. 3.85. Liver hydatid cyst with breach of the diaphragm

Fig. 3.86. Liver hydatid cyst: hydatid sand (very rare)

Differential Diagnosis

The differential diagnosis varies with the type of echographic pattern and the organ affected. In endemic countries, types II and III are characteristic of hydatid cyst, and types I and V are suggestive of hydatid cyst. However, there are alternative diagnoses:

Type I
    Cyst (biliary, ovary, mesenteric, pancreatic)
    Hematoma
    Reduplication cysts
    Metastasis, teratoma

Type II
    Abscess
    Foreign bodies

Type III
    Caroli disease
    Cystadenoma, cystadeno-carcinoma (Fig. 3.87)
    Cystic lymphangioma
    Renal cystic mass

Fig. 3.87. Pancreatic hydatid cyst mimicking a cystadenoma

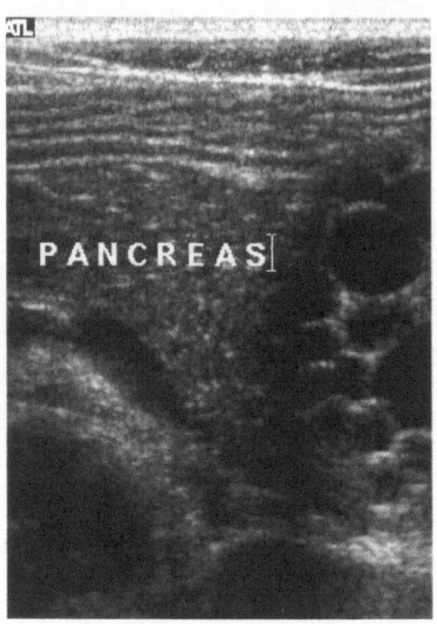

Type IV
   Abscess
   Solid tumor
   Hematoma
Type V
   Postoperative calcification
   Abscess
   Hematoma

Management of Hydatid Cyst

Surgery remains the treatment of choice for hydatidosis. However, in approximately 16% of patients, surgery may be dangerous or impossible due to post-surgical recurrence, diffuse disease, or massive peritoneal dissemination.

These situations are frequent in endemic areas and are principally due to the late discovery of the parasitosis. In addition, the hopes born with the discovery of benzimidazole compounds as a possible medical cure for hydatidosis are fading, as the reported rate of successful treatment is no more than 9–16%.

Consequently, a new interventional technique was proposed by the Tunisian Gargouri team, called PAIR:

P = puncture of the cyst under ultrasound guidance, A = aspiration of the hydatid fluid, I = injection of scolicide, sodium chloride hypertonic solution, or alcohol into the cystic cavity, and R = reaspiration of the solution without drainage, under medical treatment protection (Fig. 3.88). Other scolicide drugs, such as alcohol, have been used with good success, with or without drainage.

After PAIR, ultrasound controls showed a progressive decrease in the cyst volume and posterior wall enhancement, an increase in cyst echogenicity, and an increase in density at CT.

The involution time is variable, from 2 weeks to 2 years. Repeated PAIR procedures may be performed without complication, in order to accelerate the process of cyst involution. However, the PAIR results also depend on the cyst location. In the liver, the decrease in size occurs slowly; a minimum of 6 months is needed.

In the peritoneum, the size reduction is very fast, averaging 2 weeks. During PAIR, no anaphylactic shock and no secondary dissemination have been encountered in our experience; however, death may exceptionally occur.

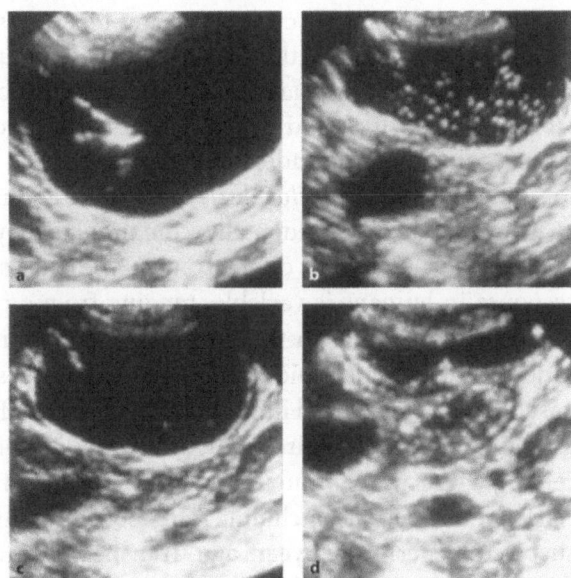

Fig. 3.88. Liver hydatid cyst treated by PAIR: **a** needle inside the cyst. **b** scolicide injection of hyperosmolar saline solution. **c** after injection. **d** after reaspiration

A moderate and short allergic reaction, with fever, may occur, but these can be easily controlled medically.

Morbidity of the PAIR method seems to be acceptable. Its cost is low, and hospitalization is much shorter than for surgery.

Negative hydatid immunologic tests cannot be considered to be a solid proof of the effectiveness of the PAIR method: it needs a total evacuation of hydatid material. There may be recurrence in 0–4% of the cases.

PAIR, today, is accepted and recommended by WHO as a good alternative for the management of hydatid cysts, but some strict rules must be respected. Today more than 4000 PAIR procedures have been done around the world; only one death was reported.

3.3.7.2
Alveolar Echinococcosis of the Liver: Ultrasound Findings
(by Michel Claudon, Alain Gerard, Alix Martin-Bertaux)

Epidemiology
Alveolar echinococcosis (AE) is a rare parasitic disease due to the intrahepatic growth of the larva of *Echinococcus multilocularis*. The disease is usually found in Central Europe, Turkey, Iran, the Soviet Union, China, Japan, and North America.

The normal parasitic cycle associates foxes, or sometimes cats or dogs, in the bowel of which the worm becomes mature, and rodents which are infested by eating plants contaminated by stools containing eggs. The larvae reach the liver and induce a tumor-like process. The parasitic cycle starts again when the rodent is caught and eaten by a fox. Up to 75% of foxes may carry *E. multilocularis* in endemic countries.

Humans can be accidentally contaminated by ingestion of infected berries or plants or by direct contact with foxes. However, the hepatic response in humans is variable, ranging from a prompt healing without any detectable lesion to the progressive development of a large hepatic process. Various epidemiological screening studies, using serological tests based on enzyme-linked immunosorbent assays (ELISAs) and ultrasound examination, have confirmed that only 0–25% of subjects with positive serologic tests were found to present abnormal ultrasound images.

Hepatic resections, including right lobectomy and segmentectomy, were successfully performed years ago. Transhepatic drainage of dilated biliary ducts or of large necrotic collections have also been found useful. However, the prognosis of the disease has changed significantly during the

last decade, due to the impact of medical treatment based on Mebenda-
zole and Albendazole. Continuous, long-term treatment (even lifelong)
has proven to be well-tolerated and effective, as lesions showed stability
in 97% of the cases. Surgery may still be indicated in the case of a limited
lesion.

Pathology

In contrast to *E. granulosus, E. multilocularis* grows with external vesicula-
tion, surrounded by a fibroinflammatory reaction (Fig. 3.89). The result is
an infiltrative tumor-like mass that very slowly invades the liver, especially
the portal spaces and hilum, the hepatic veins, and the vena cava. Microcalcifications and central necrosis are frequent, due to vascular involvement
and ischemia. Extrahepatic extension through the diaphragm or toward
the duodenum and retroperitoneum is possible, as are metastases to the
lung, brain, or bone.

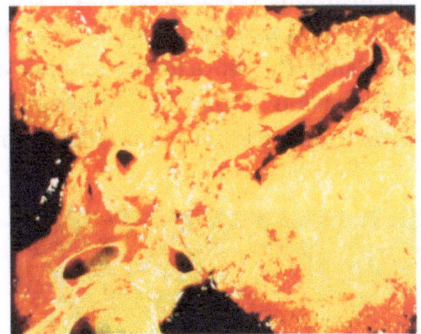

Fig. 3.89. Pathology specimen. The mass
appears as an infiltrative process, involving the main portal branches and the biliary tract

Examination Technique

Preparation is not required. The examination is initiated with a longitudinal scan to the left of the midline, demonstrating the left liver lobe,
anterior to the aorta. The transducer is moved to the right in short steps
to visualize the lobe segments anterior to the vein cava, continuing across
the interlobular area and the right liver lobe to the segments bordering
on the right kidney. The subcostal oblique scan is useful to demonstrate
extension within the right lobe.

Due to the frequent extension of the disease to the portal veins and biliary
tract, particular attention should be taken in the evaluation of the hilum

and the main portal branches, using if necessary intercostal or subcostal oblique scans, and Doppler techniques. In the case of portal hypertension, the examination should also include the spleen, the splenic and superior mesenteric veins, and the areas where porto-caval anastomoses could be demonstrated (patent paraumbilical vein, large gastric veins, or spleno-renal collaterals). Intraperitoneal fluid is nowadays rarely noted.

Pathological Findings
Hepatomegaly is frequently encountered, mostly due to the parasitic mass itself, or sometimes to the secondary hypertrophy of normal adjacent parenchyma.

There is one lesion in most cases, but sometimes multiple lesions or miliary form can be found. The right hepatic lobe is more often involved than the left one.

Several patterns of lesions can be described on sonography. Most lesions are hyperechoic, with necrotic areas and clusters of small, diffuse calcifications (Figs. 3.90, 3.91). Other presentations include hypoechoic masses and massively calcified atrophic lesions. It seems that the older is the lesion, the more heterogeneous and calcified it is.

Extension to the hilum or hepatic vein convergence is frequently found, with resulting biliary duct dilation or portal hypertension. Color Doppler

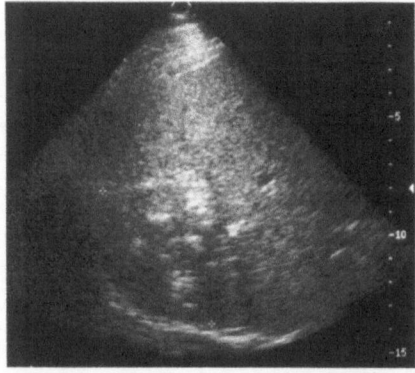 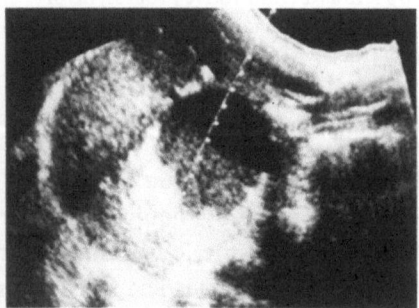

Fig. 3.90. The ultrasound examination reveals a 7-cm-diameter mass located in the right hepatic lobe, mainly hyperechoic with small clusters of microcalcification

Fig. 3.91. Large necrotic mass of the left hepatic lobe (segment 4), with fluid-debris level, and a hyperechoic peripheral rim containing calcifications

Fig. 3.92. The subcostal approach reveals a large mass, developed from the left lobe, containing several cystic areas, and having close contact with the hilum. The color Doppler mode shows the patency of the portal vein

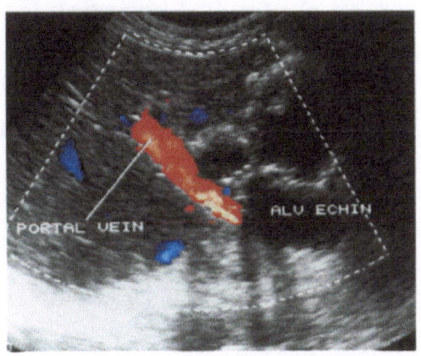

may be helpful to demonstrate patency of involvement of the main vessels (Fig. 3.92). Lymphadenopathy is rare.

Differential Diagnosis

Because of the tumor-like appearance of the parasitic process and the potential of multiple lesions, the differential diagnosis includes mainly hepatocarcinoma and metastases. Other entities to be discussed are hepatic abscess and benign tumors. However, the frequent presence of clusters of microcalcifications (90%) is of great value in suggesting the diagnosis, especially if there are few clinical symptoms and/or suspicious history (e.g., rural life). The diagnosis can be easily confirmed by serological tests, which are of high sensitivity and high specificity.

Pitfalls, Alternative and Supplementary Methods

CT scan is very helpful because it can better demonstrate areas of microcalcification. T2-weighted MR images are more effective than US and CT in showing cystic or necrotic areas, giving a grape-like pattern. Both imaging methods are required to make a precise evaluation of intra-and extrahepatic involvement of the disease, which is difficult in the far field by sonography because of the marked attenuation of the ultrasound beam throughout the fibrous and calcified parasitic tissue.

Diagnostic Efficiency

Ultrasound is a very useful technique to detect hepatic involvement by AE, in large screening studies in endemic areas, or in selected patients. Serological tests are an easier way to confirm the diagnosis than percutaneous biopsy. CT scan and/or MRI are required for a better evaluation of the extension of the disease, and for the follow-up under medical treatment.

CHAPTER 4

Ultrasound Features in Childhood Infection

IBTISSEM BELLAGHA · WIEM DOUIRA · AZZA HAMMOU ·
HASSEN A. GHARBI

In medicine, it is obvious that children are not young adults. At this age, the diseases are mainly different: some diseases are characteristic of the structure of their growing organs, others are congenital malformations. In this chapter, we will discuss some diseases in which ultrasound (US) can play an important role, even in developing countries. Osteomyelitis is a good example; US is a useful tool to diagnose the early stage of this affection. Transfontanellar US is also very useful in the study of meningitis (including early and late complications).

4.1
Ultrasound in Osteomyelitis

Acute hematogenous osteomyelitis still constitutes a diagnostic and therapeutic challenge. Infection almost always occurs by hematogenous colonization of growing bones by bacteria, usually *Staphylococcus aureus*. The metaphysis is usually the site of seeding. The onset of acute osteomyelitis is typically rapid and progressive.

Early clinical consideration, confirmation, and treatment are essential to prevent or minimize morbidity.

Osteomyelitis usually affects a single bone. Sites of predilection of acute infection are the fast-growing and large metaphyses around the knee, wrist, and shoulder. Flat bones are affected in 25% of the cases.

Clinical presentation of pediatric osteomyelitis is a temperature increase, local pain, soft tissue swelling, redness, and tenderness to palpation. Usually, a history of recent local trauma is found, but infection in neonates and infants can be clinically silent.

Once clinical suspicion is aroused and the physical examination and laboratory tests are in keeping with an infectious process, plain film radiographs should be obtained, because they may provide clues for other pathologic conditions. The earliest sign in osteomyelitis is the deep soft tissue swelling. Further swelling involves the muscles and the superficial subcutaneous soft tissues. Bone destruction and periosteal reaction may be obvious, but only 10 to 21 days after the onset of the disease. At that stage, antibiotic therapy should be established.

Bone scintigraphy using Technetium 99m methylene diphosphonate lends itself to the localization of the inflammatory process in osteomyelitis, but without any specificity. Increased vascularity of hyperemia and initial bone resorption allow concentration of the isotope at the focus of acute infection.

Echography must be done as soon as possible, before the antibiotic therapy is established.

The earliest sign of osteomyelitis is nonspecific soft tissue swelling adjacent to affected bone. The most characteristic ultrasonic feature is a subperiosteal fluid collection contiguous with the bone.

The US examination should look for more than 2-mm elevation of the periosteum by a hypoechoic or anechoic zone tapered in the two ends located usually in the metaphysis (Figs. 4.1, 4.2). The subperiosteal fluid

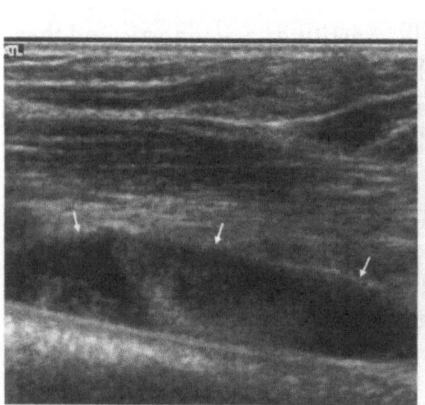 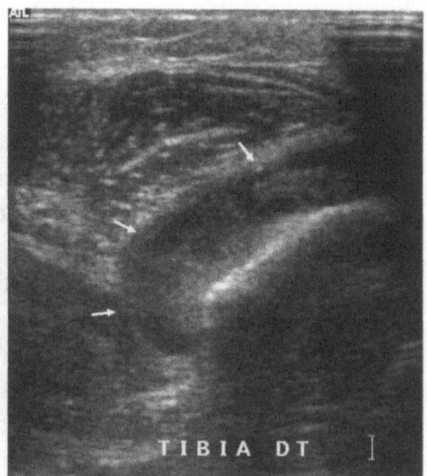

Fig. 4.1. Sonography of acute osteomyelitis of the humerus. Coronal scan depicts echogenic subperiosteal fluid in the metaphysis (*white arrows*)

Fig. 4.2. Sonography of acute osteomyelitis of the right tibia. Transverse scan depicts echogenic subperiosteal fluid (*white arrows*)

collection never crosses the physis; one of the two ends stops close to the growth plate.

An ultrasound examination is not complete until the whole circumference of the paraosseous tissues is explored. The adjacent joint should be explored in order to detect contiguous joint effusion .

In some difficult areas such as the elbow, the hand, or the foot, US examination of the contralateral limb may help to distinguish subtle findings.

Although a diagnosis of osteomyelitis cannot be established on the basis of demonstration of such fluid collection at US, the main role of US lies in the performance of immediate US-guided fluid aspiration or drainage by an interventional radiologist or, better, surgical drainage, which drains the subperiosteal fluid and the intraosseous fluid almost always found in the medullary space.

When the initial study is not positive, radiography and US exploration must be repeated regularly, at best daily, until the subperiosteal fluid collection appears.

An ultrasound examination with normal results does not exclude bone infection; correlation with clinical findings, laboratory data, and results of other imaging modalities is always indicated.

CT and MR imaging are not screening methods, but are very useful in detailing the osseous changes and the soft tissue extension of osteomyelitis. Although MR imaging is the most often performed modality in acute osteomyelitis, the availability, speed, and low cost of sonography make this technique attractive, especially in centers that encounter problems of access to the other imaging modalities.

4.2
Ultrasound in Brain Infection in Neonates and Infants

Brain infections remain frequent in some developing countries. Early recognition of central nervous system infections in children is extremely important, as the long-term effects upon the brain may be devastating.

Congenital Infections The manifestations of the infection differ, depending upon the age of the fetus at the time of infection and the bacterium. In general, infections during the first two trimesters will result in congenital malformations, whereas those that occur during the third trimester are manifested as destructive lesions.

4.2.1
Cytomegalovirus

Congenital cytomegalovirus disease is one of the most frequent infections among newborns. Generally, the virus is transmitted to the fetus by the transplacental route; if so, neurologic and developmental abnormalities are common.

Some newborns have various hematologic, neurologic, and developmental symptoms and signs including hepatosplenomegaly, microcephaly, impaired hearing, and small head size. Other infants develop neurologic or developmental abnormalities in the first year of life.

US can show:

- punctured intracranial periventricular calcifications in the basal ganglia and in the subcortical and cortical regions
- multiple, bilateral subependymal cysts
- hyperechoic images within the basal ganglia
- Ventricular dilatation may be present, with enlargement of the subarachnoid spaces.

4.2.2
Toxoplasmosis

Toxoplasmosis is a transplacental fetal infection by *Toxoplasma gondii*. In the first trimester, fetuses are less infected, and neurologic lesions are very important; 65–80% of the fetuses are infected in the third trimester, but with an asymptomatic benign disease.

In newborns, the neurologic signs are hydrocephalus, chorioretinitis, abnormal cerebrospinal fluid, and seizures. The US findings are large ventricles, hydrocephalus, periventricular and cortical calcifications, and areas of porencephaly.

4.2.3
Herpes Simplex Virus

Most cases of herpes simplex virus (HSV) result from the exposure of the fetus to maternal type II herpetic genital lesions as the baby passes through the birth canal. Symptoms usually develop within a few days or few weeks. The principal clinical findings are neurologic symptoms such as focal or generalized seizures, ocular signs, lethargy and visceral disease with skin lesion, jaundice, respiratory distress, and hemorrhage.

There is no early specific US sign, but within 3 days, patchy widespread hyperechoic areas in the white matter and the cortical gray matter are seen. Later on, US can show large punctuate or gyriform subcortical or periventricular calcifications (usually bilateral) and ventricular dilatation.

Diffuse cerebral atrophy evolves with encephalomalacia.

4.2.4
Congenital Rubella

A fetus is infected with congenital rubella by the transplacental route. The earlier the fetus is infected, the more serious are the neurologic lesions. Cataracts, glaucoma, cardiac malformation, hearing loss, and psychomotor retardation occur when the infant is infected during the first trimester. The clinical presentation at birth is usually one of lethargy, hypotonia, a large or bulging fontanel, cataract, and microphthalmia; irritability and seizures may develop after a few months.

US findings are:

– ventriculomegaly secondary of marked loss of brain tissue
– hyperechoic areas with calcifications of the white matter and the basal ganglia.

4.2.5
Meningitis

Bacterial meningitis is the most common form of central nervous system infection in children. The diagnosis of meningitis is made from clinical signs and symptoms and the results of a lumbar puncture.

US findings in bacterial uncomplicated meningitis are usually normal. Occasionally, good visibility of a cortical fissure or echoic subarachnoidal fluid can be obtained.

Complications of meningitis can be diagnosed by US:

– Ventriculitis: hyperechoic ependyma, ventricular dilatation (Fig. 4.3), abnormal echoes within the ventricular fluid, loculation of cerebrospinal fluid (Fig. 4.4) within the ventricles
– hydrocephalus,
– hyperechoic heterogeneous areas in the brain (Fig. 4.5)

Fig. 4.3. Sonography of meningitis with increase in the skull perimeter. Transverse medial scan depicts ventricular dilatation and an echoic heterogeneous aspect of the brain and cerebellum parenchyma (*white arrows*)

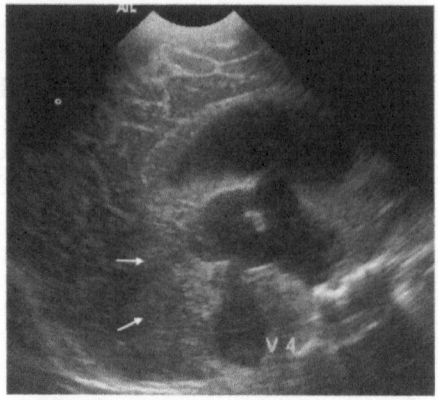

Fig. 4.4. Sonography of meningitis: loculation of intraventricular cerebrospinal fluid

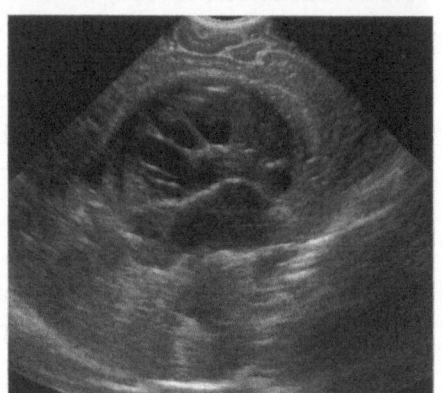

Fig. 4.5. Sonography of complicated meningitis. Transverse scan of the brain depicts a heterogeneous hyperechoic aspect of the brain with ill-defined white matter/gray matter

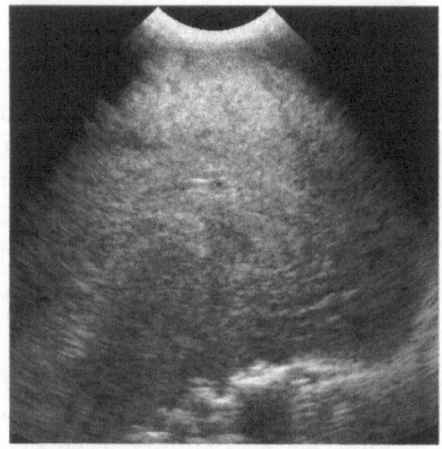

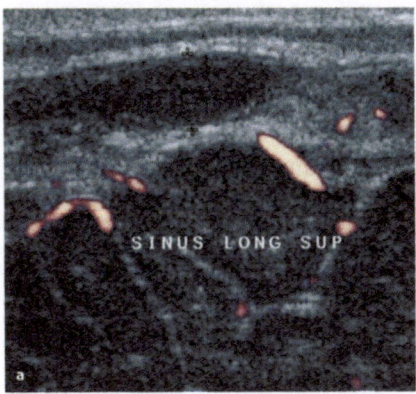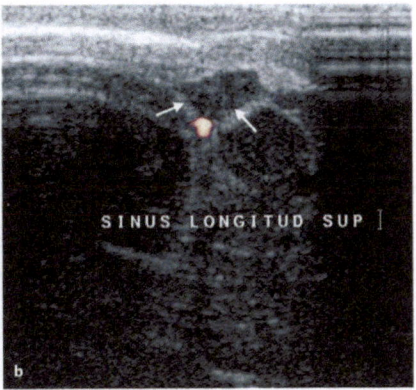

Fig. 4.6a,b. Doppler sonography of acute meningitis with neurologic symptoms. Transverse (**a**) and coronal (**b**) scans from the anterior fontanel shows the superior sagittal sinus thrombosis without flux inside the sinus (*white arrow*)

– Sinus thrombosis: hyperechoic aspect within the sinus, without any flux in the color Doppler (Fig. 4.6); in that case an MRI should be performed.

4.2.6
Encephalitis and Brain Abscess

Encephalitis and brain abscess can develop as complications of meningitis. Cerebritis is the earliest stage of purulent brain infection. It is a focal or multifocal suppurative process that may resolve, or evolve to frank abscess formation.

At the cerebritis stage, brain sonograms can reveal a widespread hyperechoic area with irregular borders within the white matter close to the ventricle. Differentials are ischemic or hemorrhagic lesions, but with different clinical presentation.

Later, US shows a well-defined area with small hypoechoic images. Mild to moderate mass effect is present.

At the cerebral abscess stage, sonography depicts a complex cystic pattern with an echoic wall and a sonographically hypoechoic or mildly hyperechoic central zone of necrosis. When the abscess is not large, a target-shaped lesion can be seen with three layers: hyperechoic peripheral, hypoechoic inside, and a central very hyperechoic area. At this stage, the mass effect has usually decreased.

4.2.7
Viral Encephalitis

Many viral infections involve the central nervous system. It is very difficult to differentiate among most viral infections based on radiologic or clinical criteria. The clinical presentation is usually fever, alterations in consciousness, and seizures. The US findings in these patients are a patchy area of hyperechogenicity and a poor differentiation of white matter and gray matter.

4.3
Ultrasound in Abdominal and Gastrointestinal Infections

US shows no specificity in children. Like adults, children can be affected by hepatic or splenic infection as abscesses or tuberculosis or parasitic infection (e.g., hydatid cyst).

Appendicitis has the same US criteria in adult and children.

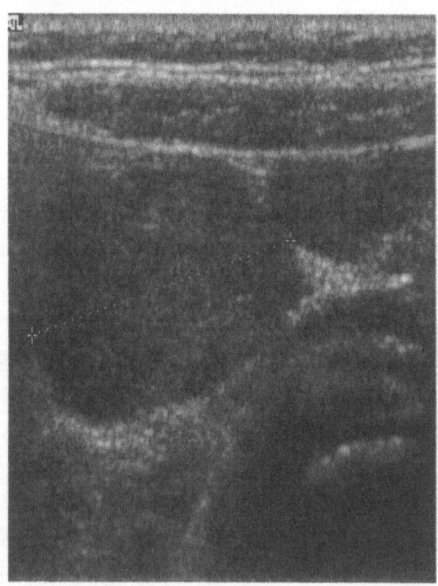

Fig. 4.7. Abdominal sonography of the right iliac fossa in a child with abdominal pain: nodal enlargement

A specific presentation is observed in children: mesenteric lymphadenitis. This is a viral mesenteric lymph node infection that has nearly the same clinical presentation as appendicitis, but with a normal white count. Sonography with a high-resolution linear array probe depicts multiple node enlargement (more than 1 rightiliac fossa (Fig. 4.7), with a normal appendix.

Glossary

Absorption: Direct conversion of (ultra)-sound energy into heat; leads to reduction of ultrasonic intensity in biologic tissue and indicates a cause of possible hazards (see Chap. 1, Sect. 1.5)

Acoustic enhancement: Relative intensification of the echoes distal to areas causing an attenuation below average (*"sonolucent"* areas), especially fluid collections, due to a relative excess of time-gain compensation

Acoustic shadow: Echo-free or relatively echo-poor (partial shadow) area on the ultrasonic image occurring distal to interfaces, causing a total reflection of the ultrasound (gas, foreign bodies), or structures causing relatively high *attenuation* (bones, fibers)

Acoustic streaming: Movement of fluid due to ultrasound (demonstrated as movement of the echoes arising within a nonhomogeneous fluid)

Anechoic, anechogenic: Denotes an absence of (internal) echoes, typically for fluid (better echo-free)

Artifacts: Features in an ultrasonic image that are not referrable to real structures with regard to shape, intensity, or location

A-scan: One-dimensional technique; each echo causes a vertical deflection of the electron beam on a display proportional to its intensity; used for measurements

Attenuation: Intensity loss of ultrasound in the tissue due to *absorption*, reflection, and *scattering* measured in decibel per centimeter

Axial resolution: The ability to distinguish objects in the direction of the ultrasound beam emitted by a transducer

B-scan: Mode of display in which echoes are presented as light spots on the screen

Cavitation: Formation of voids in a molecular structure during the negative-pressure phase of an (ultra)-sound wave

Color Doppler technique: *Duplex technique* with the Doppler signals displayed as colored pixels, depending on their mean velocity

Contrast agents: Encapsulated *microbubbles* used intravenously to enhance the Doppler signal from streaming blood

Contrast harmonic imaging: Based on the technique to receive only the echoes with a doubled frequency (2nd harmonic) compared to the fundamental (emitted) frequency. This technique enables a better differentiation of the signals caused by the contrast agents, because microbubbles produce a much stronger 2nd harmonic signal than tissue

Coronal plane: A plane corresponding to the long axis of the body, but at right angles to the *longitudinal (sagittal) plane.* (e.g., a coronal scan may be obtained with the transducer placed on the side)

Coupling agent: A gel or liquid used to obtain close contact of the surface of the transducer with the skin, without air bubbles interfering with the ultrasound transmission

Crystal: Polar crystals are used as ultrasound *transducers* for converting electrical energy into ultrasound waves, and vice versa

Curved array: *Transducer* with the arrangement of two or usually more *crystals* on a convex surface

Decibel (dB): Unit of measure of acoustic energy

Depth gain compensation (DGC): Used as a synonym for *time gain compensation (TGC)*

Display: Visual presentation of echoes

Doppler effect: The original (emitted) frequency is changed when it strikes an *interface* moving toward or away from the transducer

Doppler frequency: Describes the difference between original (emitted) and received *frequencies*

Duplex technique: Fixed combination of a Doppler system with the B-scan image

Echoes: Reflected ultrasound signals that form the basis for diagnostic ultrasonography

Echo-free: Denotes an absence of (internal) echoes, typically for fluid (syn.   *anechoic*)
Echo pattern: Describes the intensity and distribution of all echoes of a certain area (organ or tumor)

Echo-poor: Describes an *echo pattern* consisting of few and weak echoes

Echo-rich: Describes an *echo pattern* consisting of many strong echoes

Far field: That part of the ultrasound field distal to the *focus*

Focus: The natural focus is the narrowest point of the ultrasound field between the near and far fields

Focusing: Adjustment of the ultrasound beam to a particular distance (depth), to obtain the best resolution in the region of interest

Frequency: Number of complete (ultra)-waves per second

Gain: The relationship between energy output and input in an amplification system, expressed in decibels

Hertz: Unit of frequency measurement equal to one cycle per second

Hyperechogenic (hyperechoic): Synonym for *echo-rich*

Hypoechogenic (hypoechoic): Synonym for *echo-poor*

Impedance: Resistance to an acoustic wave

Impedance jump: Sudden change ("jump") in acoustic wave resistance at the interface between two materials (tissues) with different acoustic properties

Intensity: Acoustic energy per unit area

Interface: Technically a part interposed between two structural components to compensate for their imperfect fit

Lateral resolution: The (poorer) resolution in a direction transverse to the ultrasound beam

Linear array: The linear arrangement of two or more *crystals* in one line, which are activated electronically in groups

Longitudinal scan: A plane corresponding to the anterior-posterior long axis of the body

Mechanical index (MI): A number indicating the relative risk of an adverse bioeffect resulting from a mechanical effect, such as cavitation, during an ultrasound examination

Microbubbles: See *contrast agents*

Mirror effect: Total reflection of the ultrasound pulses by some structures, e.g. the air-containing lung

M-mode: Continuous tracing of the ultrasound echoes for the evaluation of moving structures (echocardiography). Synonyms: M-scan, *TM-scan*, time motion

Near field: The part of the ultrasound field between the *transducer* and the *focus* (synonym: Fresnel zone)

Parallel scan: Two-dimensional B-scan with the single ultrasound beams running parallel (typical image of linear array transducer)

Phantom: A device for testing or calibrating ultrasound equipment

Piezoelectric effect: Property of *polar crystals* to convert mechanical energy (pressure and tension) into electrical energy (= ultrasound receiver) and vice versa (reverse piezoelectric effect = ultrasound transmitter)

Pseudocavitation: Release of gas in aqueous solutions by means of ultrasound

Pulse-echo techniques: Term for those (i.e., most) ultrasound techniques in which the ultrasound is emitted in very short pulses and the returned echoes are analyzed

Real time: A B-scan technique with a fast construction of images (around 15 / sec), creating the impression of a continuous image

Resolution: See *axial* and *lateral* resolution

Reverberation: Reflection of ultrasound between two nearly parallel surfaces back and forth repeatedly. The repeated echoes arrive at the transducer with a delay and are positioned in the image in a doubled or multiple distance

Sagittal scan: Corresponds to *longitudinal scan*

Scanning plane: The plane in which the two-dimensional ultrasound beams are scanned into the body or organ, and from which the echoes are received

Scattering: The reflection and refraction of an ultrasound beam nondirectionally by a reflector smaller than the *wavelength*

Sector-scan: Two-dimensional B-scan produced by diverging ultrasound beams (typical for mechanical real time and curved array transducers)

Sonolucent: Term describing tissues and structures with a low (below average) *attenuation* of the ultrasound

Spectral Doppler: Display of all *frequencies* of the Doppler signal over time

Specular reflector: Reflectors (tissue surface or vessel wall) with a smooth surface and a diameter greater than the diameter of the *wavelength*

Stimulated acoustic emission: The destruction of the microbubbles by ultrasound (high *MI*) creates a very short but strong signal used, e.g., for the differentiation of liver tumors

Thermal index: A number indicating the maximum internal temperature elevation that might occur during an ultrasound examination

Time gain compensation (TGC): Electronic amplification of the echoes depending on their distance from the *transducer* (synonym *depth gain compensation, DGC*)

Tissue harmonic imaging: B-scan technique based on analysis and image construction using echoes with a doubled fundamental frequency (second harmonic) exclusively

TM-scan: Synonym for *M-mode*

Transducer: A device that converts one form of energy into another (here electric energy into mechanical ultrasound waves and vice versa)

Transverse scan: Scanning plane right angled to the long axis of the body

Ultrasound: Mechanical pressure waves beyond the upper limit of the human hearing (i.e., > 20,000 Hz)

Wavelength: The length of a single cycle of the (ultrasound) wave. It is inversely proportional to the *frequency*.

Suggested Reading

General Ultrasound, Pediatric Ultrasound, Intervention

Barcovich AJ (1996) Pediatric neuro-imaging, 2nd edn. Lippincott-Raven, New York

Bianchi S, Martinoli C. (2005) Ultrasound of the musculoskeletal system. Springer, Berlin Heidelberg New York (in press)

Buscarini L, Campani R (2001) Abdominal ultrasound. Idelson-Gnocchi, Naples

Buscarini E, Di Stasi M (1996) Complications of abdominal interventional ultrasound. Poletto, Milan

Cerri GG (2002)Tumores e lesoes focais hepaticas. In: Cerri GG, de Oliveira IR. Ultrasonografia abdominal. Revinter, Rio de Janeiro

Giorgio A, Tarantino L, de Stefano G, Francica G, Esposito F, Perrotta A, Aloisio V, Farella N, Mariniello N, Coppola C, Caturelli E (2003) Complications after interventional sonography of focal liver lesions: a 22-year single-center experience. J Ultrasound Med 22(2):193–205

Hennerici M, Neuerburg-Heusler D (2005) Vascular diagnosis with ultrasound. Thieme, Stuttgart 2005

Krebs CA, Giyanani VL, Eisemberg RL (1993) Ultrasound atlas of disease processes. Appleton & Lange, New York

Mathis G, Lessnau KD (2003) Atlas of chest sonography. Springer, Berlin Heidelberg New York

Meire H, Cosgrove D, Dewbury K, Farrant P (eds) (2001) Abdominal and general ultrasound. Churchill Livingstone, London

Middleton WD, Kurtz AB, Hertzberg BS (eds) Ultrasound, 2nd edn. Elsevier/Mosby

Palmer P (ed) (1995) Manual of diagnostic ultrasound. WHO, Geneva

Ultrasonic Diagnosis of Infectious and Parasitic Diseases

Acquatela H, Schiller NB (1980) M-mode two-dimensional echocardiography in chronic Chagas' disease. Circulation 62:787–798

Akata D, Ozmen MN, Kaya A, Akhan O (1999) Radiological findings of intraparenchymal liver Ascaris (hepatobiliary ascariasis). Eur Radiol 9(1):93–95

Bartholomot G, Vuitton DA, Harraga S, Shi Da Z, Giradoux P, Barnish G, Wan Yh, MacPherson CN, Craig PS (2002) Combined ultrasound and serologic screening for hepatic alveolar echinococcosis in central China. Am J Trop Med Hyg 66:23–29

Bureau NJ, Chhem RK, Cardinal E (1999) Musculoskeletal infections: US manifestations. Radiographics 19:1585–1592

Cerri GG, Alves VAF, Magalhães A (1984) Hepatosplenic schistosomiasis mansoni. Ultrasound manifestations. Radiology 153:777–780

Cerri GG, Barros N, Magalhães AEA (1990) Radiologic study of Chagas' disease. In: Bigot JM, Moreau JF, Nahum H, Bellet M (eds) Radiology. Elsevier, Amsterdam, pp 145–156

Cerri GG, Oliveira IRS, Machado MM (1999) Hepatosplenic schistosomiasis. Ultrasound evaluation update. Ultrasound Q 15:210–215

Caremani M, Maestrin R, Benci A (1995) AIDS-related cholangiopathy: sonographic evaluation of a sample of HIV patients. Mediterranean J Infectious Parasitic Dis 2:73

Choi BI, Han JK, Hong ST, Lee KH (2004) Clonorchis and Cholangiocarcinoma: etiologic relationship and imaging diagnosis. Clin Microbiol 17(3):540–552

Choi D, Hong ST, Lim JH, Cho SY, Rim HJ, Ji Z, Yuan R, Wang S (2004) Sonographic findings of active Clonorchis sinensis infection. J Clin Ultrasound 32(1):17–23

Dreyer G, Santos A, Noroes J, Amaral F, Addiss D (1998) Ultrasonographic detection of living adult *Wuchereria bancrofti* using a 3.5 MHz transducer. Am J Trop Med Hyg 59:399–403

Dreyer G, Dreyer P, Piessens W (1999) Extralymphatic disease due to bancroftian filariasis. Braz J Med Biol Res 32:1467–1472

Dreyer G, Noroes J, Figueredo-Silva J, Piessens FW (2000) Pathogenesis of lymphatic disease in bancroftian filariasis: a clinical perspective. Parasitol Today 16:544–548

Gharbi HA, Hassine MW, Brauner MW, Dupuch K (1981) Ultrasound examination of the hydatid liver. Radiology 139:459–463

Gargouri M, Ben Amor N, Ben Chehida F, Hammou A, Gharbi HA, Ben Cheikh M, Kchouk H, Aaychi K, Golvan JY (1990) Percutaneous treatment of hydatid cysts (*Echinococcus granulosus*). Cardiovasc Interv Radiol 13:169–173

Hatz C, Jenkins JM, Ali QM (1988) Morbidity associated with Schistosoma mansoni infection as determined by ultrasound: a study in Gezira, Sudan. Am J Trop Med Hyg 39:196–201

Hong ST, Park KH, Seo M, Choi BI, Chai JY, Lee SH (1994) Correlation of sonographic findings with histopathological changes of the bile ducts in rabbits infected with *Clonorchis sinensis*. Korean J Parasitol 32:223–230

Jeffrey RB (1988) Gastrointestinal imaging in AIDS: abdominal computerized tomography and ultrasound. Gastroenterol Clin North Am 3:507

Lim JH, Ko YT, Lee DH, Kim SY (1989) Clonorchiasis: sonographic findings in 59 proved cases. Am J Roentgenol 152:761–764

Marchetti F, Piessens FW, Medeiros Z, Dreyer G (1998) Abnormalities in the leg lymphatics are not specific for bancroftian filariasis. Trans R Soc Trop Med Hyg 92:650–652

Marin-neto JA, Bromberg-Marin G, Pazin-filho A, Simões MV, Maciel BC (1998) Cardiac autonomic impairment and early myocardial damage involving the right ventricle are independent phenomena in Chagas' disease. Int J Cardiol 65:261–269

Moraes FJ, Moraes TA, Felix VN, Pereira-Barreto AC, Betarello A (1988) Esophageal manometry and vectorcardiography staudy of asymptomatic patients with Chagas' disease. Rev Inst Med Trop S Paulo 406–410

Noroes J, Addis D, Santos A (1996) Ultrasonographic evidence of abnormal lymphatic vessels in young men with adult *Wuchereria bancrofti* infection in the scrotal area. J Urol 156:409–412

Noroes J, Dreyer G, Santos A (1997) Assessment of the efficacy of diethylcarbamazine on adult *Wucheria bancrofti* in vivo. Trans R Soc Trop Med Hyg 91:78–81

Oloveira LCM, Nascimento RS, Rocha A, Goncalves EG, Silva JMF, Oliveira VA, Ferreira RMS, Buso AG. Colelitiase em chagasicos cronicos. Arq Gastroenterol 34:222–226

Oudjane K, Azzouz M (2001) Imaging of osteomyelitis in children. Radiol Clin North Am 39:2

Palmer P, Reeder MM (2001) The imaging of tropical diseases, 2nd edn. Springer, Berlin Heidelberg New York

Paranagua-Vezozzo D, Cerri GG (1992) Duplex haemodynamic evaluation of hepatosplenic mansoni schistosomiasis. Mem Inst Oswaldo Crus 87:149–151

Rang NN (2003) An ultrasound scoring for prediction of developing shock for Dengue hemorrhagic fever. Ultrasound Med Biol 29 [5 Suppl]:189–190

Reeders JWA J, Goodman PC (2001) Radiology of AIDS. A practical approach. Springer, Berlin Heidelberg New York

Reuter S, Nussle K, Kolokhytas O, Haug U, Rieber A, Kern P, Kratzer W (2001) Alveolar liver echinococcosis: a comparative study of three imaging techniques. Infection 29:119–125

Schulman A (1998) Ultrasound appearances of intra- and extrahepatic biliary ascariasis. Abdom Imaging 23(1):60–66

Setiawan MW, Samsi TK, Wulur H, Sugianto D, Pool TN (1998) Dengue haemorrhagic fever: ultrasound as an aid to predict the severity of the disease. Pediatr Radiol 28(1):1–4

Simao C (1981) Chagas' disease. In: Reeder MM, Palmer PES (eds) Radiology of tropical disease. Wilkins & Wilkins, Baltimore

Smith FJ, Mathieson JR, Cooperberg PL (1994) Abdominal abnormalities in AIDS: detection at US in a large population. Radiologo 192:691

Teixidor HS, Godwin TA, Ramirez EA (1991) Cryptosporidiosis of the biliary tract in AIDS. Radiologo 180:51

Thulkar S, Sharma S, Srivastava DN, Sharma SK, Berry M, Pandey RM (2000) Sonographic findings in grade III dengue hemorrhagic fever in adults. J Clin Ultrasound 28(1):34–37

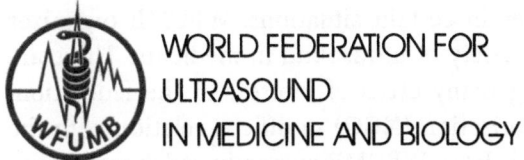 WORLD FEDERATION FOR
ULTRASOUND
IN MEDICINE AND BIOLOGY

WFUMB is a federation of affiliated organizations consisting of regional
federations and national societies. The regional federations cover national
societies of ultrasound in Europe (EFSUMB), in Asia (AFSUMB), in Latin
America (FLAUS) and in Africa (MASU). The national societies are North
America (AIUM), and Australasia (ASUM).

Presently the total number of individual members is 49,581, compris-
ing physicians, scientists, engineers and ultrasonographers. EFSUMB has
16,178 individual members from 25 European countries. AFSUMB has
15,487 members from 12 Asian countries. AIUM has 7295 members from
the United States, 232 from Canada and 856 members from other countries. FLAUS has 6070 members from 12 countries in Latin America. ASUM
has 2531 members from Australia and New Zealand, and MASU has 932
individual members from 31 African and Mediterranean countries.

Objectives (article 3 of the constitution): "The objectives of the Federation shall be scientific, literary, and educational. Its aims shall be to
encourage research in the field; to promote international cooperation in
the field; and to disseminate scientific information. In pursuit of these
aims the Federation may, in the relation to its specific field of interest, en-
gage in the following activities: sponsoring of meetings; publication of an
official journal and other official documents; cooperation with other societies and organizations in specific learning; appointment of commissions
on special problems; awarding of prizes and distinctions. It may promote
the formation of national or regional societies or groups, the coordina-
tion of bibliographic and informational services and the improvement of
standards in terminology, equipment, methods and safety practices, and
generally shall promote improved communication and understanding in
the world community using ultrasound in medicine and biology."

WFUMB organizes world congresses in ultrasound every three years
covering the whole field of diagnostic ultrasound. WFUMB sponsors

other congresses and courses in certain situations. WFUMB organizes and sponsors workshops on safety of ultrasound in medicine. There are various committees covering many areas of interest to the federation. As a non-governmental organization (NGO) in official relation with the World Health Organization (WHO), WFUMB currently collaborates with the WHO on various education programs by organizing and sponsoring courses and working for the creation of educational centers and education and reference material. The official journal of WFUMB, *Ultrasound in Medicine and Biology* (UMB), is published monthly by Elsevier Science Inc. *Echoes*, the WFUMB newsletter, is published twice a year and distributed to members of affiliated organizations.

Subject Index